Nursing Care: From Theory to Practice

This book is dedicated to Carole and Mark, two very supportive
and caring colleagues without whom this book would
not have been written.

Nursing Care: From Theory to Practice

by

CHRIS BASSETT RN, BA(HONS), RNT
University of Sheffield

W
WHURR PUBLISHERS
LONDON AND PHILADELPHIA

British Library Cataloguing in Publication Data

A catalogue record for this book
is available from the British Library.

ISBN 1 86156 431 7

Typeset by Adrian McLaughlin, a@microguides.net
Printed and bound in the UK by Athenæum Press Ltd, Gateshead, Tyne & Wear.

Contents

Preface

This book explores the essence of nursing care. It is part of a personal journey that I began as a new student nurse at the age of 21. This journey has involved experiences and observations of nursing care at many levels. The journey has seen me (the author) in the varied roles of 'hands-on student nurse carer', then as staff nurse, then as 'expert supervisor' (senior staff nurse) of care, this leading to a 'facilitator of care' (charge nurse) and most recently as a 'teacher of care' (nurse lecturer) in a school of nursing. My interest in care and caring as experienced by the nurse remains just as strong as it did as a student. Why and how do nurses care? My interest now is mixed with experiences and insights, gathered over 20 years or so. This book aims to increase insight into how nurses care for patients. Unsurprisingly, I suppose, the early pages of this book seem to be made up of a long list of questions. I just hope that by reading the book you will find at least some of the questions will be answered!

At the age of 21 I became a pupil nurse. (Pupil nurse training has now been discontinued in the UK. It was the less academic route to professional nursing.) I entered pupil nurse training as I had no educational qualifications from school (I failed the entrance test), and this was the only way I could become a nurse. That said, I always enjoyed nursing and found particular satisfaction in working with patients and their families. However, from my earliest time in nursing, I was interested in why nurses nursed, what nursing care actually was and how nurses made sense of and understood their relationship with the patient. Again from my earliest times in nursing, nurses who were able to form a strong caring relationship with patients always impressed me. Those nurses seemed to be more effective in what they did in terms of nursing care. I feel that I was effective in this way with the patients. I was also interested in nurses who did not seem to easily form effective caring relationships with patients; I wondered why this was, as to me caring was the key part of nursing and *not to care* was *not to nurse*.

Throughout my nursing career I became more aware of the apparent strength that caring brought to the nurse. I progressed through nursing, moving from staff nurse in a medical ward to staff nurse in intensive care and then on to charge nurse in intensive care. All through this time questions relating to the fundamental question of what nursing care really meant kept coming back to me.

In recent years I have been a lecturer in nursing studies and have in many ways been reminded of and carried back to my own early years in nursing. It has been extremely interesting to meet and teach newcomers to nursing, and in doing so I have gained further insights into healthcare providers' motives, views and attitudes towards the caring acts and key issues in nursing. It is only now in writing this book that I am exploring the motives, attitudes and beliefs of nurses relating to their perceived roles and responsibilities in nursing.

Chris Bassett

CHAPTER ONE

Why do nurses do what they do?

Introduction

My personal position in relation to care and caring in nursing is closely aligned with that of Madeleine Leininger (1981), who states that the words 'nursing' and 'care' are synonymous. She proclaims, 'Caring is nursing' and that 'Caring is the central, unique, dominant, and unifying focus of nursing.'

Why study care?

Why worry about the meaning of care? How will a better understanding of care help nurses to do their jobs better? The answer to these questions must be that, if one is interested in the future of nursing and believes in promoting the unique and therapeutic role that nurses can play in the lives of patients, we need to know more about this, arguably, vitally important part of our role. This view is strongly supported by Leininger (1978), who believes that a systematic study of caring phenomena can yield important information in the development of nursing science. This study is an exploration of care as perceived by nurses. It is aimed at gaining a deeper insight and understanding into the acts and motives of the care and caring provided by nurses.

Norris (1989) holds a similar view, stating that caring is expected to change theories which guide practice, foster research which tests theories and modify nursing practice. Furthermore, nursing does not stand still: it does not exist in a vacuum, and it is becoming more important to more people worldwide. Health and healthcare are becoming extremely valuable commodities; they are also becoming more and more expensive, particularly in the developed world. It is vital that we develop a clear understanding of care in order that nursing can develop and fulfil the important role that it provides.

However, Castledine (1998) points out, rather worryingly, that the word 'nursing' seems to be slipping from use in the National Health Service today; instead we have healthcare trusts referring to their medical, surgical and general prowess.

Why choose nursing?

Many people worldwide opt to become nurses. Why might this be? When one considers the pressures and tasks nurses have to perform, it may be worth pausing to explore this question in more detail. Could it be that by considering reasons and motives for nursing we may gain a further understanding and insight into what nurses value about the act or role of caring? A common comment that is widely made from all quarters is that nursing is a vocation. This view or perception strikes me as having echoes of a religious calling. This term 'vocation' may be described as a preordained course for one's life.

In the literature, there are some commentators who follow or at least align themselves with the vocational school of nursing motives. Lane (1987) offers an analysis of nursing care as being, for some nurses, a 'calling'. She states that this process occurs in three main ways. First of all, the person called views the profession through a different lens. Nursing for them has a deep, personal and religious or humanitarian meaning; this factor helps the nurse to reach out more compassionately, more hospitably and more sensitively to the patient. Secondly, nurses can be more aware of the effect that they will have on the other person. Associated with this is an inner reflection that will help the nurse elucidate more clearly the struggles heard from within the patient. Finally, the nurse becomes more aware of the meaning of partnership: a partnership of what Lane calls, 'the source of all healing'. Lane, who is clearly both a committed Christian and also a nursing academic, concludes her paper with the statement, 'What more noble vocation can we experience in nursing than that of committing our whole lives to the care of the spirit in our patients and in ourselves? This is what makes us truly human and completely committed nurses.'

The concept of nursing as a vocation is certainly an interesting and clearly deeply held view and, as such, must be respected. It is my belief, however, that for the majority of nurses working in the modern healthcare system the idea of a calling or vocation is one that is not understood in these, at times, strongly religious terms. It would appear that the relatively modern concepts of 'professionalism' and 'career' are not really compatible with that of vocation or calling. The question therefore remains: what are the motives for caring in the majority of nurses that practise today? Is there a relationship between the 'called' nurse and the 'professional' nurse?

Raatikainen (1997) carried out a study to explore this very issue. She describes a calling as 'a deep internal desire to choose a task or profession which a person experiences as valuable and considers her own. She devotes herself to the task and strives to act according to its highest principles. The aim of a calling task is to serve people altruistically.'

Raatikainen wanted to find out if there was a difference between nurses who experienced a calling and those who did not. She used a questionnaire that compared the nurses who considered themselves as having an experience of being called with those nurses who did not. The questionnaire measured the levels of nurses' knowledge concerning their patients' needs, motivations and values, nursing action and collaboration between nurse and patient. The results appeared to show that nurses who experienced a calling described themselves more often than other nurses as having a greater knowledge or 'feel' for their patients' physical condition, psychological state and general needs. Despite some limitations identified in the research method, the researcher concludes that the so-called 'calling' appears to be a strong resource for the nurse. Raatikainen suggests that nurses who have a vocational bent are more effective in the way they care for their patients. This concept is intriguing and would certainly benefit from further exploration.

A factor missing from Raatikainen's research is the notion of being paid to work as a nurse. What of the majority of nurses who currently practise? Do they experience a calling? All of the nurses who are known to myself are paid to nurse and need to work. At this point it may be beneficial to consider whether or not the concept of paid care affects one's motive to nurse and care; the first thought must be 'yes'. It certainly seems to undermine the notion of vocation or calling. However, in the real world, all or most of us need to earn money. But it is true to say that there are many other occupations from which to choose and which are often better paid and with better prospects.

Raatikainen's research outlined above does not provide insight into any motives for becoming a nurse. However, it does provide important evidence and insight into what nurses themselves perceive to be important personal qualities related to the practice and process of caring for patients.

Care and caring

In her seminal work, Leininger (1988a) states that human caring is a universal phenomenon with culture affecting the way that caring expressions, processes and patterns are exhibited. The nursing profession by its nature is not in fact a single group as perhaps might at first be imagined by an outsider; it has numerous individual groups and subcultures, such as children's nurses, psychiatric nurses, intensive care nurses, theatre nurses and so on. Each group is given an individual identity by differing work areas, technical skills and unique traditions and languages. Of course, to suggest that nurses are the only group involved in healthcare that cares would be quite wrong; families, lay carers and volunteers expend a great deal of time and effort caring for those in need. However, as Brycynska (1997) points out, the nurse's way of conceptualizing care is different from others, such as the lay public. Nursing care, it can be argued, is the result of an ongoing moral development tempered by the personal and professional aspects of socialization, both primary and secondary.

The public have high expectations of nurses; they expect that the nurse will care and be caring towards them or their loved ones. The notion of care is reflected in their code of conduct (NMC 2002). Nurses are bound by this code, and, if it is proven that nurses do not abide by the code in their professional lives, they can be removed from the register. The code underlines the responsibility of the job and the fact that nurses' patients may be harmed or even die if they do not do their job properly. Nursing is a very responsible job. Nurses are there, on call and caring all of the time for the patient, protecting their life, while doctors are with patients for a comparatively short time.

What is care?

The first stop on the journey begs the question, 'What is care?' Despite the increasing volume of nursing study, it is perhaps surprising that the literature as it stands is still reasonably limited in the number of available studies which explore the essence of care. This is surprising, as nursing must surely be based upon the foundation of care and caring. Roach (1991) takes the argument one step further and states that 'when we cease to care, we cease to be human'. Could it be that, as Radsma (1994) points out, 'if nurses cease to care, do they cease to be nurses?'

It is my belief that nursing and care are intimately related. However, strangely enough, the subject of care and caring within nursing is laden with complexity and assumption. Everyone uses the words 'care' and 'caring' every day in many situations. Allmark (1995) highlights the fact that these words are very frequently used in differing ways and contexts. As a noun, 'care' can mean worry or anxiety. It can mean some sort of safe haven, as in 'putting someone into care'. As a verb, it may describe where the attitude of care is primary: 'I care'. Or, if 'I am caring' is used, it suggests a judgement about what kind of person someone is. Norris (1989) suggests that words in common use, such as 'care', can be problematic: the common meaning does not change because the word is adopted by or identified with one particular group, such as nurses.

'Caring' can have a very personalized definition. It quite possibly means different things to each individual nurse. There is clearly a close association between the above terms. Nurses and nursing use all of the above meanings to help describe what they do and what it is that makes the nurse's intervention special. Stevenson (1990) equates the term 'nursing care' with clinical interventions. This view, however, may be limiting in that it describes what a nurse might do in terms of physical activity, but it does little to expand our true understanding of the motive of the nurse. It is, in my view, important to be clear about motives. Why do generally healthy, often young, individuals surround themselves with the elderly, the sick and dying, handling shit, spit, vomit and blood? Is there a personal need or calling? Is it for the money?

Why worry about gaining a better understanding of care? What is there to be gained on embarking on a quest for insight other than as part of a purely academic exercise? Does it matter as long as nurses continue to provide expert nursing skills to our patients? As Cheung (1998) points out, if caring is indeed the essence of nursing, the nurse's own interpretation of caring must have relevance for their nursing practice. One way of clarifying the concept of caring is to examine the nurse's own interpretations of caring.

In some ways a nurse's role is to protect the patient from the doctor: on several occasions I have often queried a doctor's orders in medication or fluid therapy and in so doing have prevented harm being done to the patient. In addition to this, a large part of nursing practice involves explaining to the patient surgical or medical treatment modalities, comforting them and providing human tenderness, supporting the patient and their significant others through often frightening and confusing processes. This is why we need to explore the motives and definitions of care so that nurses can continue to help patients survive their treatments both physically and psychologically. Leininger (1984) maintains that 'Care remains a major way to legitimise nursing and make its unique contribution to humanity known to the public.'

There is a lot written by academics on caring, but the real truth about caring must surely come from nurses themselves. That is why I asked nurses to describe and discuss what nursing meant to them. This is where the real insights come from and these parts of the book bring home the, often harsh, realities of care.

The respondents

Fifteen qualified nurses from a variety of backgrounds were interviewed. I asked them in their own words to explain what caring means to them. In addition to the fifteen experienced nurses, six student nurses were also

invited to participate in the interviews. They too were interviewed individ-
ually and asked to discuss issues surrounding care from the perspectives of
relative newcomers to the profession of nursing. Many moving and insightful observations and statements were made that add important parts to the
picture and allow glimpses of what it means to care from both a student
nurse's point of view and their more experienced qualified-nurse colleagues. The participants' biographies can be found in the appendix at the
end of this book.

Finding out about care

How did the nurses share the information in this book? The nature of the
way that nurses interpret their role of care and caring, despite increasing
academic study, is still not clear. It is agreed by many nursing scholars that
the concept of care and caring is an inherently difficult notion to clarify.
However, it is clearly important to explore the experience and perceptions
of nurses that underpin their personal philosophies of care and caring. Of
course, as with any inquiry, it is the way that that exploration is undertak-
en which is the key to its success. How should we go about understanding
difficult issues such as care?

The phenomenological approach

The approach taken in this book to make clear the views and beliefs of the
nurses interviewed uses the lived, expressed experiences of real nurses. It
is called 'phenomenology'. Don't worry, though. I will not cover this
research method in great detail. However, it is important to quickly look at
how the themes were arrived at.

Research given the label phenomenology is interesting because it spans
a wide variety of methodological approaches, theoretical underpinnings
and disciplinary associations. It is heavily influenced by sociological and
anthropological research in which descriptive, interpretive aspects are
major ideals. As such it explores the feeling and beliefs of individuals
involved in the caring experience. Heidegger (1962) believes that experiencing the world around us is the same as caring for it. He writes of how
care gives meaning and rhythm to all experience. In order to understand
as fully as possible the ways that nurses understand care, it is important to
explore the 'life worlds' of the nurses. Drew (1989) suggests the life world
consists of the 'social, practical, experiential and taken-for-granted dimension' that can be frequently overlooked by researchers, particularly those
who come from a quantitative perspective. Phenomenology is therefore

the study of phenomena or the appearance of things. In phenomenological study an attempt is made to understand another person's subjective experiences and feelings by studying their field of expression. The field of expression is made up of speech, expression, gestures and intonations (Bassett 1994b). Language is used to convey information and to describe reality. Words are the building blocks of everyday reality (Holstein and Gubrium 1994); it is the words of the nurses here in this book that are used, following interpretation, to provide insights into care.

This book will not, however, dwell on the methodology. Instead it will explore in some detail the actual emotions and beliefs of the nurses. In doing so we will see that there are many ways that nurses see their caring role. For those interested, there are many good books and articles that explain the research method; these are included in the references section at the end of this book.

Choosing the nurses

The first group of nurses comprised fifteen qualified nurses who were colleagues or were undertaking educational courses at the university department where I work. They were asked to participate in an individual, informal and loosely structured guided discussion lasting approximately 30 minutes that would be recorded, transcribed and analysed following the discussion. They were known to be interested in caring issues and had often spontaneously shared insights relating some of the fundamental issues of nursing practice, and seemed to hold strong views on caring, which they were ready to share. I explained well before the interview what the study was about. I told them I wanted them to explain what care meant to them. In addition, I prepared them by showing them the questions I was going to ask them, and in particular I drew attention to the final question (this last question gave them the opportunity to describe a situation from their practice that epitomized a caring situation).

The student sample

Apart from *qualified* nurses I wanted to understand how *student* nurses saw care as well. The students who were recruited comprised six members: two from the first year, two from the second and two from the third year of the advanced diploma in nursing course. This stratification was carried out to enable consideration of possible changes to views and attitudes over the three-year education process of the students. The following themes emerged:

- making a connection
- encouraging autonomy
- giving of oneself
- taking risks
- supporting care
- emotional labour

These themes provide the later chapters in the book and are at times funny, disturbing or sad, but always fascinating.

CHAPTER TWO
What is care?

Introduction

This chapter explores some of the literature that aims to provide us with insights into the definition of the concepts surrounding care and caring. Shultz et al. (1998) point out that caring, as a uniquely nursing domain, has been discussed and debated since the time of Florence Nightingale; yet in reality it still remains a poorly defined concept in nursing practice.

The concepts of care and caring are inherently difficult to define. This is certainly clearly reflected in the existing literature. Valentine (1991) states that the conceptual domains for the phenomenon of caring have not been fully defined, and we have no universal meaning or definition of caring, or the caring performed by nurses in a healthcare setting.

It is important that we as nurses understand care and caring and incorporate them into our nursing theories. According to Eddins and Riley-Eddins (1997), nursing theory is to be properly thought of as situation producing, with an aim for activity (that is, applied to actual practice). I fully accept this view, as it is my personal view that any nursing theory should be developed with the specific aim in mind that it would ultimately enhance patient care, as the whole point of nurses surely is to provide care for patients!

Perhaps the lack of a comprehensive definition of caring is due to the elusive, subjective and imprecise nature of caring itself. The terms 'care' and 'caring' are part of nursing's ideals, actions and underlying philosophy (Leininger 1981, Watson 1988). They are, however, as McKenna (1993) states, historically intertwined with tradition, and, if caring is indeed the essence of nursing, nurses' own interpretation of caring must have relevance for their nursing practice. That is why I wanted to ask nurses what they thought. However important caring is, as Radsma (1994) states, until Leininger began to systematically study care in the 1950s, very little time or real effort had been spent exploring the foundation and meaning of care in nursing.

Caring, according to Swanson (1991), is a nurturing way of relating to a valued other towards whom one feels a personal sense of commitment and responsibility. It is only in the past 20 years or so that a systematic and rigorous study of the concept of caring has been carried out. It is only with the outstanding work of notable nursing academics such as Gaut (1983), Roach (1987), Watson (1988), Benner and Wrubel (1989) and Swanson (1991), to name but a few, that care and caring have been better, though by no means comprehensively, understood. Despite the steady increase in the number of studies, there appears to have been no significant increase in the shared understanding of what exactly care might be; arguably, quite the opposite may be the case. Indeed, Webb (1996) states that to say there is still a lack of consensus about the definition of care is a major understatement.

Tschudin (1986) outlines a key issue of the caring relationship as applied to the nurse. She sees caring as geared to the other person in a relationship – in the nurse's case, the patient. The patient may be different from the nurse, culturally, physically or philosophically. Despite these differences, the nurse has an obligation to provide care for the patient; this is highlighted in the nurse's code of conduct (NMC 2002). The nurse has to provide care for the patients in an unbiased way, without prejudice or favour.

When considering care and caring in nursing, there are specific issues that we need to consider, most important of which perhaps being the motives for caring and ultimately how one might better assist the patient throughout their illness in an increasingly technological age, where humanity is arguably being pushed to the periphery of healthcare. Sprengal and Kelley (1992) see the ethics of care as being a basis for holistic care. They believe that the current interest in the ethics of care has grown as the technology in, and the depersonalization surrounding, healthcare has increased.

One popular view of the nurse today might be as a 'super knowledgeable' technician making vital decisions, operating complex and important equipment, adjusting gases, balancing fluids and drugs, helping maintain a patient's – sometimes dodgy – grip on life. This is true in many areas today of nursing care, but these, albeit important, skills can be carried out without the nurse really and truly being in a caring relationship, or can they? Sprengal and Kelley surmise that caring is an intrinsic characteristic of humankind, and as such the capacity to care is a prerequisite of ethical behaviour. That being the case, ethics and caring are inseparable entities. Allmark (1995) poses a counter view. In his argument, he states that caring is not good in itself but only when that care is expressed in the right way. He identifies two aspects of care: cognitive and emotional.

1. Cognitive: when someone cares about something they see as of concern, interest or value to them. To care about something is to believe it to be good.
2. Emotional: the attachment of care is betrayed by a whole set of emotions and emotional dispositions. The emotions may include anger or sorrow at what one cares about being treated unfairly, or feeling pity, compassion, joy or contentment at their care.

His points, which are sound when applied specifically to the general public may, however, be a bit shaky when related to nursing care and caring or, indeed, any of the professional caring services. This is because nursing, medicine in general, social work etc. are all bound by stringent ethical codes relating to their practice, at least in the United Kingdom. The concept of care is a key part of the nurse's, midwife's and health visitor's code of conduct; the first of its sixteen clauses states that nurses should act at all times in such a way as to promote and safeguard the well-being of patients or clients (NMC 2002).

Care: some points of view

Care is a complex issue surrounded by questions and few answers. Swanson (1991) poses these questions:

1. Is caring a process observable only in the context of two people relating?
2. Is it embedded in the behaviour of a caregiver?
3. Or is it a perception identifiable only through the eyes of a caregiver?
4. Can caring be taught?
5. Is it a moral ideal?
6. Or is it a way of being in the world?

At this stage, let's pause again and ask the question: Is a definition of caring possible and is it even desirable? On the first point, as caring is such a complex issue that encompasses such a huge range of issues and underpinning factors, how can we, by consulting and observing nurse carers and reading the thoughts of a few dusty old nursing academics, gain a definition? On the second point, perhaps to define and measure something might spoil it somehow. To reduce caring into a series of documented steps or stages might be to seriously mess up the real power of care.

So perhaps it is not surprising that the complex phenomenon that we call 'care' is widely accepted as being a very difficult concept to define. As is usual in these situations, we turn to the dictionary to define or explain these words, care and caring, but again, as usual, the definitions offered really do not adequately express their true meanings. There are many different attempts in the literature of nursing to define care and caring; some are, of course, better than others. Watson, in her theory of human care (1979), cites ten primary 'carative factors' as forming a structure for understanding the nursing science of caring:

1. the formation of a humanistic-altruistic system of values
2. the instillation of faith/hope
3. the cultivation of sensitivity to one's self and to others
4. the development of a helping, trusting relationship
5. the promotion and acceptance of the expression of positive and negative feelings
6. systematic use of the scientific problem-solving method for decision-making
7. the promotion of interpersonal teaching/learning
8. the provision for a supportive, protective and/or corrective mental, physical, sociocultural and spiritual environment
9. assistance with the gratification of human needs
10. the allowance for existential and phenomenological forces

Eddins and Riley-Eddins (1997) see Watson's theory of caring as being primarily concerned with health promotion rather than with the specialized treatment of disease; this they consider as being essentially the domain of medicine. This is, in fact, the care/cure split, the tension between process (the nurse's preoccupation) and outcome (the doctor's preoccupation). It is true, however, that in reality the nurse (particularly today) has feet on both sides of the care/cure gap, as indeed the doctor probably has as well. Eddins and Riley-Eddins expand on Watson's universal view on caring in the following way:

1. Caring has existed at all times and in every society.
2. Caring takes place inter-subjectively.
3. Caring is related to the satisfaction of human needs.
4. Caring is respectful of human choice as to the best course of action to be undertaken.
5. Caring accepts a person as he/she is, and envisions what a person may become.
6. A science of caring is complementary to the science of curing in that it integrates biophysical knowledge with the knowledge of human behaviour to generate or promote health.

Sourial (1996) believes that care is a subjective human process, where a high value is placed upon the caring relationship between the nurse and the recipient of care. Gaut (1983) clearly states that the concept of caring has a very special place in nursing discourse. Gaut explores the concept, looking at the language and words used in care, then, taking the senses of caring derived from normal usage, she tries to identify possible new senses of caring.

Considering the use of words in care, she outlines the three general senses of caring:

1. attention to or concern for
2. responsibility for or providing for
3. regard, fondness or attachment

Gaut's subsequent review of nursing's scholarly literature verified the assumption that 'caring', despite its common usage, lacked the clarity and preciseness essential to underpin scientific endeavour. In the final step, Gaut asks the simple question: 'What must be true to say that nurse S is caring for patient X?' This, Gaut felt, would provide the framework for the logical conditions that must be met to call any action a caring action. She finally proposed three conditions that instigated a caring action.

1. Nurse S must have knowledge about patient X to identify a need for care and must know that certain things could be done to improve the situation.
2. Nurse S must choose and implement an action based on that knowledge and intend the action as a means for bringing about a positive change in patient X.
3. The positive change condition must be judged solely on the basis of a 'welfare for patient X' criterion.

Gaut, later on (1993), identifies that the exploration of the subject of caring is gaining ascendance and can be seen as a new, important and unifying basis for nursing science. As such, it is considered as essential that further widespread, creative exploration is required as this will generate new ideas, insights and ways of thinking about caring, nursing practice and research. This has certainly been the case in recent years as nurse theorists continue to explore the issues surrounding nursing care.

Madeleine Leininger must be considered along with Jean Watson as being amongst the leading nurse theorists exploring care and caring in nursing. Leininger had undergone doctoral training in anthropology, and combining this academic discipline with a nursing background enabled her to consider nursing and the basis of nursing in new and exciting ways. She felt strongly that patients had to be cared for in a culturally sensitive way – an approach today that is considered as obvious and essential. However, before her work, cultural individualization and holism were not widespread in nursing curricula or practice. During the progress of Leininger's work on caring, not surprisingly, her definitions developed over the years.

In 1970, care was first defined in its noun sense as being 'the provision of personalised and necessary services to help man maintain his health state or recover from illness' (Leininger 1970). As a verb Leininger believed it implied a 'feeling of compassion, interest, and concern for people'. As her work progressed, she explored the differences between caring and curing; she believed that caring was the most critical component of the curing process (Leininger 1977). She came to consider that without caring there could be no curing but that there could be caring without curing; this important theme has persisted throughout her writing to the present day. Leininger was also amongst the first nurse theorists to compare generic caring with professional caring. Generic care she defined as being 'those assisting, supportive, or facilitative acts toward or for another individual or group with evident or anticipated needs to ameliorate or improve a human condition or life way' (1981). Professional caring was defined as 'those cognitively learned humanistic and scientific modes of helping or enabling an individual, family, or community to receive personalised services' (1981).

By the early 1980s, Leininger had become a leading light of the idea that nursing and care were synonymous. 'Caring is nursing,' she proclaims. 'Caring is the central, unique, dominant, and unifying focus of nursing.' She continues to explore care and caring and is considered today as a highly influential and important researcher and nursing scholar.

Swanson (1991) attempts to define care by exploring nursing in three perinatal contexts in which she spoke to lay and professional carers and their patients. From these interviews she created five behavioural categories of caring:

- knowing
- doing for
- being with
- enabling
- maintaining belief

Swanson (1991) offers us the example of caring as 'being with'. A woman who was undergoing dilatation and curettage describes the action of her nurse: 'He tried to be as gentle as possible. He even cried a bit. He made me feel like he cared.' The tears were seen as evidence that he cared about her. However, as Phillips (1993) points out, it may be that, had the nurse omitted a necessary procedure in an attempt to spare the patient pain, he would have not given successful care irrespective of his intentions, emotions or the perceptions of the patient. Morse et al. (1991) consider that there are five ways in which caring might be conceived:

1. as a human trait, that is, as something which is naturally part of the condition of being human

2. as a moral imperative, that is, as a fundamental virtue or value
3. as an affect, that is, extending oneself towards one's patients and beyond one's job description
4. as an interpersonal interaction, that is, as something which exists between one person and another
5. as a therapeutic intervention, that is, something which is deliberately planned with a goal in mind

They conclude that caring had been studied as a human trait, moral imperative, affect, interpersonal relationship and nursing therapy. It is my belief that it is important, if not vital, that study into care and caring does not become just an academic exercise but contributes in a meaningful way into how nurses understand and deliver care to their patients. That is what I hope this book is really about.

Castledine (1998) describes his view of the caring process in the following way. Caring should not be confused with wishing well, liking, comforting, maintaining or simply having an interest in what happens to another. It is not an isolated feeling or a momentary relationship, nor is it simply a matter of wanting to care for a person. Caring is something special; it is a process, a way of relating to someone; it needs to develop in the same way that a friendship develops only over time. He identifies the key elements of nursing care as:

1. knowing yourself and the value of nursing to humanity
2. sensing, perceiving and experiencing that there is someone or a group that needs you
3. experiencing the intensity of the relationship that will stimulate you to carry on your work
4. having the knowledge and skill to be of help to the person or group, this element being what differentiates nursing from caring

Kyle (1995) believes that caring is a complex phenomenon involving more than a set of caring behaviours. It is a process including moral, cognitive and emotional components, which are culturally derived. Waddell (1996) points out that caring is often associated with weakness, passiveness, nurturing or perhaps a codependent type of relationship. She also believes that nurses need to develop their own individual meaning of what caring is to them. She seems to reject much of the philosophical preoccupation related to defining care. Instead, she appears to make care a very practical issue, which is an approach that appeals to myself, being practical and dynamic by nature. By caring, she means that we are willing to exert effort to help others in an active and practical nature.

Conclusion

Perhaps a true definition of care is not possible; care and caring can arguably be considered as an individual concept. Despite the increase in studies by nursing scholars into caring theory, the debate has not really progressed past the descriptive phase. In reality the academics have, as usual, probably muddied the waters somewhat. What we as a profession, however, do need to do is to greatly increase our understanding by asking what care means to both nurses and patients alike. In achieving a deeper understanding of these important concepts of nursing care we can further shape and guide nursing forward, and, in doing so, we will increase the potential to improve the quality and focus of the care that we provide our patients.

CHAPTER THREE

What nurses and patients think care is

Introduction

This chapter explores the literature surrounding how nurses and patients understand and perceive the terms 'care' and 'caring'. Here some very interesting insights can be seen in the studies into what care and caring are. It is obviously very important to compare how nurses and patients view care, because, if we don't give patients what they want, we sure ain't giving them a good service!

Caring and nursing

Few could argue that caring is not an integral part of the nature of nursing. Leininger (1986) states that caring is the essence of what nursing is. Many, including myself as stated earlier, would not disagree with this view and would argue that to try to nurse without caring is not in fact nursing. Scott (1995) points out that healthcare nurses have a strongly recognized role and, as such, are totally required to care for patients without question. This is supported by the nurses' code of conduct (NMC 2002).

In order to push the care debate further, it is essential to explore the way nurses interpret and perceive their roles as caregivers. A majority of articles and papers on the subject of care and caring begin with a lengthy description of how caring is the central and unifying feature of nursing. Jensen (1993) defines care as being a state, or mode of being, that resists command and instruction. As stated earlier, care is a difficult entity to explain or define. It is a prime example of emotion, thought and action coming together to provide comfort, both physical and emotional, for another individual. Caring is considered by many as the primary task of nursing (Staden 1998); indeed, it is argued by some commentators as being 'the fundamental human imperative that must be obeyed by all of humanity' (Gordon 1991).

Caring obviously has a physical manifestation; it also has a psychological, spiritual and social existence. Perhaps the public's view or perception of the nurse is most often that of physical carer, helping the patient eat, drink, wash or even helping them through the dying process. Some nurses, in my experience, are also of the view that caring physically is primarily what nursing is. They would describe this as 'real nursing'; indeed, it is a standing joke in some quarters of the profession that psychiatric nurses are not real nurses, as they don't actually do anything (patently not true, of course).

James (1992) states that it is the provision of physical care that defines the nurse's caring role. Without doubt, nursing has always had a strong practical focus. This is still the case, as nursing and particularly general nursing requires the acquisition of lots of very practical skills needed to help the patient get by.

So what do nurses really think caring is?

Dyson (1996) carried out a study aimed at eliciting nurses' views of caring attitudes. The participants, nine in all, were all hospital nurses, and several significant themes emerged. These included 'consideration and sensitivity', 'honesty and sincerity', 'general approach' and 'giving of oneself'. All of the above characteristics underline the importance of the human aspect of care within the caring process.

She found that caring, as seen by the participating nurses, involves a combination of what the nurse does and what the nurse is like as a person. The participants felt that nurses should show consideration and sensitivity. They also felt that nurses should make time for patients and appear unhurried and in control (not always easy to do today).

Coulon et al. (1996) carried out research to explore the meaning of what 'excellence in nursing' means to nurses themselves. They sent questionnaires to students in their first year of study and to registered nurses who had previously qualified. Responses revealed that at all times the patients were at the centre of the nurses' concern. They felt that professional practice, delivered both competently and holistically, was the key to care for the patient and their family.

Professionalism, it was felt, underpinned all aspects of nursing-care delivery. It implied that quality and high standards were expected. *Holistic care* means that by adopting a certain approach to patients, encompassing the psychological, social, emotional and spiritual needs of the patient, the nurse should provide an individualized package of care to the patient. The theme *practice* relates to the implementation of competent and exceptional nursing care. Many nurses believed that excellence in nursing care involved the awareness and implementation of the latest and best evidence of knowledge and skills. Interestingly, the first-year students attached more importance than the other, more experienced nurses to personal traits in the delivery of excellent nursing care. Managerial and organizational skills were also considered as being important to excellent nursing care.

Rittman et al. (1997) asked oncology nurses what skills and attributes they used in caring for their patients. They were asked to write about an experience that taught them something about what it means to care for a dying patient. Themes were taken from the narratives in the following ways:

Knowing the patient and the stage of illness: it was seen as a key factor that the nurses must gain knowledge of the patient, for with this comes the ability to understand the trajectory of the disease. A 'special' bond may or may not occur between the nurse and patient. The achievement of a close bond could provide strength for both patient and nurse. However, even without the close bond, 'good' nursing care was still given. A mark of expertise in oncology care was considered as being able to accompany the patient and their family throughout the course of the illness leading to death. Nurses described the decision to become involved with patients and that this could enhance the nursing care which could be given to the patient. However, they also stated that it could be damaging to the nurse, especially if they had had a painful or difficult experience with a similar patient in the past. Some of the nurses particularly valued the quality of physical care of the dying patient and saw it as an entrée to providing emotional care. Caring for the physical body provided nurses with a way of knowing the patient which would be impossible without the intimacy of seeing, touching and caring for the body. As patients allow nurses access to the most private parts of their physical being, they trust and open themselves to sharing their thoughts and fears. It was seen by respondents that easing the struggle is achieved through expertise in providing physical and emotional care in a seamless process.

Preserving hope: nurses spoke of the need to keep hope alive when patients were entering the final stages of life. Wherever possible, they tried to get the patient home to make the most of the time they had left. Nurses approached caring for terminally ill patients as opportunities to participate in a life event completing itself rather than only seeing the loss of shortened lives.

Easing the struggle: nurses can even ease the struggle and promote a peaceful death. It was considered as important to help family members become involved with the care of the patient. This included knowing when and how to talk to the patient's family to encourage them to be with patients while they die. One nurse described the skill of providing physical care 'smoothly, not as separate steps, not a time for physical care and a time for talking' – all carried out in an integrated way.

Providing for privacy: the cornerstone for oncology nursing was considered as being the provision of privacy while dying. Nurses described how they went to great lengths to accomplish this goal. Although privacy issues are often culturally defined, oncology nurses valued the provision of privacy highly as an important caring action.

Research has also been carried out into nurses and caring in the field of gynaecology. McQueen (1997) uses a qualitative approach to explore the verbalized experiences of twelve nurses relating to the care they provided for their patients. After analysis of the data, the following situations were identified as being of relevance to care:

Direct patient care: the relationship between nurse and patient was seen as particularly important as the nature of this type of nursing is often of an intimate and private nature. Following on from this, nurses felt that it was essential to be especially supportive, dextrous, gentle and sensitive in their approach. Nurses also believed that understanding and empathy were also demonstrated in their concern with the patients' lives beyond the hospital, such as preparations for hospital, concerns about ongoing management of the home and feelings of separation from the family during their hospital stay. Some stated that their being women helped them empathize with the patients.

Caring for patients having a pregnancy terminated: the research found that, despite having their own views about abortion, they all felt that their role was to meet the needs of all patients. Nurses also showed a clear appreciation of the mental turmoil that can accompany a termination.

Caring for patients having a miscarriage and problems with fertility: nurses exhibited the ability to show empathy and were well aware of the importance of sharing in the women's sorrow and of being there for the patient.

Caring for terminally ill patients: the nurses reported the belief that the intellectual and emotional work involved in caring for dying patients is often not openly recognized as significant caring work alongside physical care.

Caring for patients who are emotionally upset: although this area of care was often difficult to cope with and nurses found it hard to know what to say, they still believed that it was important to show compassion and empathy.

Caring for patients behind a façade: sometimes patients were waiting for important test results that nurses and doctors often knew and the patients did not. Patients would ask the nurses, but the nurses did not feel able to disclose the information before the doctor had first spoken to the patient. These kinds of situations, the nurses felt, affected honesty and trust in their caring interactions with the patients.

Caring for relatives: nurses in all areas of care deal regularly with relatives. The nurses believed that it was important to support, comfort and empathize with them as well as the patients.

Caring for the nurse: nurses believed that it was important to care for other team members. The support of colleagues and cooperative teamwork offered support for nurses in providing emotional and physical care in their work.

In summary, the nurses, in describing their work in great detail, high-lighted the importance to them of a high level of interpersonal and humanistic care for the patient in their workplace.

Critical-care nurses were included in a study by Barr and Bush (1997). Fifteen nurses were asked to describe their experiences of caring. Caring in the critical-care area was revealed to be 'a multidimensional, complex process involving assessing and addressing patients' and their families' unique needs with the goal of improving the patients' condition, and acknowledging nurses' living out of caring ways in their own lives'. Four categories were drawn from the research. These were:

1. *nurses' feelings*: characterizing this category were sensitivity, empathy, loving, general concern and genuine interest.
2. *nurses' knowledge and competence*: included in this category were knowledge of the patient, setting priorities for the patient, knowledge of the family and technical, interpersonal, expressive and listening competence.
3. *nurses' actions*: incorporated around giving physical care, communicating (speaking and listening), touching, supporting, teaching, mediating, advocating, making decisions and taking responsibility for their actions.
4. *patient and family outcomes, and nursing rewards*: occurred when the patient moved to another stage of recovery and went to different nursing units. The nurse could see relief in the patient's eyes, the patient became happy and the patient and family were satisfied.

When considering the effects of high technological input (a factor that is increasing in all areas of nursing) in the role of the critical-care nurse, a caring approach was considered as being definitely an important factor in caring for the patient. For the fifteen nurses involved in the exploration of the caring activities in their daily work, caring was seen as a series of processes consisting of an affective process, a cognitive process, an action process and an outcome process.

'The emotional labour of caring' is a concept that was defined by Hochschild (1983), meaning the undefined, unexplained and difficult component of the work, mainly carried out by women. This concept is important in several ways as it adds to the general theories of caring. It is applicable to nursing care, which is still mainly carried out by women. It also, when explored in an appropriate and sensitive way, provides a great deal of extra insight into not just what caring behaviours might be but importantly what they might mean to the nurse, and how they might affect the nurse. The general concept of emotional labour was later expanded by Bolton (2000), who developed the notion of nurses giving 'emotional gifts' to their patients. She points out that the term 'emotional labour' stresses that some of the skill of a professional carer is in creating the 'correct' emotional climate by managing emotion to the benefit of the patient. The student nurse respondents describe this 'emotional management' or control later on in my study, with reference in particular to the difficulties they face dealing with painful practice situations.

Staden (1998) explores this concept of emotional labour with three nurses; she uses a phenomenological approach in her in-depth inquiry. Through interview analysis, the data was coded into themes, which were clustered into categories. The categories are:

- private/public spheres
- appearing caring
- nurses are human (too)
- giving of yourself
- value and visibility
- coping

Private and public spheres: the women were considered as 'emotional labourers' by the researchers. They all used skills and emotional techniques learnt and practised at home in their work-based caring. It was recognized in the analysis that emotional labour was as demanding as physical labour; success was dependent on the successful handling of each situation.

Appearing caring: there was a feeling that it was essential that nurses appear caring both to the patient and to the general public. Genuineness, openness and some self-disclosure were considered important to the process of caring. However, the same respondent felt that too much caring might lead to overdependency in the patient. The way the nurse expressed herself was adjusted to fit in with the patient's mood (if the nurse was happy, she would dampen down her image portrayed on her face to be in keeping with the mood of the situation). It was concluded that nurses may need to become adept at 'deep acting', meaning to change feelings and alter outward appearance for the sake of the patient.

Nurses are human too: one of the nurses stated that relatives were sometimes surprised when nurses got attached to patients and cried sometimes when they worsened or died. It was considered important and positive by the nurses that they (the nurses) are viewed as being human and, as such, subject to emotions.

Giving of yourself: it was expressed by one of the respondents that it was a good thing to give the patients examples of emotions so that they might identify subdued emotions within themselves. Nurses are interdependent of and connected with the patient. One interesting exposure was that one of the nurses, who worked in psychiatry, felt it could be helpful to the patients by working through her own problems and in that way help heal others.

Value and visibility: all respondents in this study greatly enjoyed their work and valued the caring input into their work. They alluded to skills that they brought with them from home to work. These were described as 'basically female skills', 'organizational skills' and 'how to manipulate or influence others, even their emotions, to get what you want (or win)'.

Coping: there was a general belief that emotional work is hard work. One respondent saw nurses as being a 'never-ending storage bag, and taking on others' emotions'. Caring was seen to come sometimes from colleagues when things were too difficult to easily deal with by the nurses.

This report is of real importance in informing the theoretical debate relating to how we as nurses care not just for the patients but also for each other. The respondents saw nursing as being a highly satisfying and rewarding pastime, but it was made clear in the study that the nursing role is characterized by extreme emotional demands. This seems to be part of what it is in providing high-quality care in all healthcare situations.

Fagerberg and Kihlgren (2001) studied 20 registered nurses' experiences of caring for elderly patients. They looked particularly at positive and negative expressions of care. The nurses saw the ability to care for their patients in individualized ways as being important, but, when the patients were confused, this led to negative feelings that they were then unable to individualize the care they provided. Trust was also seen as a valued aspect of care, as was the provision of adequate numbers of skilled nurses to provide care. On a negative point, the nurses were unhappy when, owing to staffing constraints, patients received what the nurses saw as sub-standard care. Commitment was also identified as being a key aspect of care, and nurses felt unhappy about colleagues who did not show similar commitment to their care. Knowledge of the elderly and what it might be like to be old was also identified as a positive way that supported good care. Those nurses who it was felt did not have the knowledge about ageing were considered as being less able to give care. Finally, the nurses stated that the best nurses had courage to look after the patient's interests and question the physician's instructions if they felt they were not in the best interests of the patient.

What patients and nurses think care is

Larson (1984) surveyed 57 cancer patients to assess their perceptions of caring behaviours. The patients consistently ranked the highest caring behaviours as those that showed the nurse had competent and knowledgeable technical skills and abilities. Following this study, Larson (1986) measured oncology nurses' perceptions of what they thought would make the patients feel cared for. Conversely, the nurse sample revealed that it was the expressive humanistic behaviours that ranked highest, such as listening, comforting and expressing sensitivity.

Smith and Sullivan (1997) explored the perceptions of nurses and patients in a long-term care-home setting. The two groups (fourteen patients and fifteen nurses) were given identical lists of care behaviours. Nurses perceived the item 'listens to the patient' as the most important caring behaviour. Their ten highest-ranking behaviours included seven expressive behaviours (for example expressing trust, acceptance of feelings, faith etc.) and three instrumental behaviours (for example physical care, treatment etc.). Patients ranked the item 'puts the patient first, no matter what happens' highest. Of the ten highest-ranked behaviours, five were instrumental and five expressive. Two of the valued instrumental behaviours involved 'providing honest information to the patient' and treatments. Although patients did not rank 'listens to the patient' as highly as nurses, they still ranked it in the top ten. Patients included 'is cheerful' amongst their ten highest, whereas nurses ranked it 29th.

Generally, nurses and patients were in broad agreement about the importance of caring behaviours; however, it may be that comparisons are context-dependent. For example, patients in this study were all long term; therefore it might be that they and their nurses developed a closer rapport than patients and nurses achieve in other, more transient, settings. Larsson et al. (1998) compared cancer patient and staff perceptions (179 patients and 62 nurses) relating to caring behaviours. The results of this study found, for example, that patients perceived the dimension 'anticipates' as the most important, whereas nurses perceived 'comforts' to be the most important (Figure 3.1).

Dimension	Patient ranking	Staff ranking
anticipates	1	2
explains and facilitates	2	6
comforts	3	1
monitors and follows through	4	4
trusting relationship	5	5
accessible	6	3

Figure 3.1 Some important and interesting differences between staff and patient perceptions of caring dimensions (Larsson et al., 1998).

Comparing nurses' views on care

General nurses and psychiatric nurses generally have very different ways of working. Greenhalgh et al. (1998) carried out a study exploring these two groups' behaviours relating to the issues surrounding care. They were also interested as to how age, gender and qualification made a difference to caring behaviours. The findings of the study were summarized in Figure 3.2:

Dimension	General nurse ranking	Psychiatric nurse ranking
monitors and follows through	2	1
explains and facilitates	=4	2
comforts	1	3
trusts	=4	4
accessible	3	5
anticipates	6	6

Figure 3.2 Greenhalgh et al.'s 1998 comparison of general and psychiatric nurses' approaches to care.

A comparison of the views revealed similarities as well as differences in the two types of nurse. Age was also a factor: 'monitors' was ranked highest by the group aged 31–50, and of those nurses under 30 only 12% did not agree that they monitored their patients. By contrast, 27% of nurses over 51 did not agree that they monitored their patients. This study is interesting and thought-provoking, raising many issues between general and psychiatric nursing. Walsh and Dolan (1999) assessed views on caring of 156 nurses in the accident and emergency area (A&E) (Figure 3.3). They then compared A&E nurses with general nurses to explore differences in caring attitudes. The top six caring dimension categories of the A&E nurses were, in order:

Dimension	A&E nurses	General nurses
explaining a clinical procedure	=1	8
providing privacy for a patient	=1	2
being honest with a patient	3	6
listening to a patient	4	1
giving reassurance about a clinical practice	5	3
making a nursing record about a patient	6	21

Figure 3.3 Walsh and Dolan's 1999 comparison of A&E and general nurses' approaches to care.

Overall, the A&E nurses saw the relative priorities in care in a similar way as general nurses. However, they did not regard the importance of getting to know the patient as a person as high; this was also true with 'sitting with the patient'. It may be the nature of A&E units that accounts for this, with their comparatively rapid patient throughput. Again, nurse caring can be seen as a context-dependent perception that will differ from ward to ward and speciality to speciality.

Barr and Bush (1998) explored the views of fifteen nurses in the intensive care unit (ICU) setting. The nurses described factors that enhanced and reduced caring in the ICU. Four major factors were identified as being crucial to caring in the ICU. These were:

1. support
2. role-modelling
3. patient and family interactions
4. economic/bureaucratic forces

Support: support from colleagues was seen as essential to enable and support the respondents' work. There were also many comments regarding positive comments relating to care that was well carried out or difficult situations that were dealt with in an efficient way. Caring shown by colleagues was, in turn, seen as supportive in motivating the nurse to further caring actions.

Role-modelling: twelve of the fifteen nurses spoke of the importance of a role model in exhibiting caring behaviour to the nurses in ICU. They admired role models and found inspiration in them. Role models were seen to have a good attitude to their patients; they were kind, empathic and thoughtful towards patients and their families. They were very much considered as empowerers of care.

Patient and family interactions: strong feelings of caring were expressed in their statements about the need for expanded visiting hours enhancing care. Others saw encouraging families to become involved with their loved ones' care as a strong indicator of caring behaviour.

Economic/bureaucratic factors: demotivating factors were definitely seen to include economic and cost-containing measures. These were seen as necessary, but were the root cause of short staffing. Statements relating to anger, stress, hopelessness, frustration and burnout were described as reducing care in the ICU.

Yam and Rossiter (2000) surveyed ten registered nurses in Hong Kong to explore their perceptions of caring. Three categories emerged from the data. These were:

1. trying one's best in meeting clients' needs

2. demonstrating effective communication
3. providing a supportive environment

Trying one's best in meeting clients' needs meant providing the biopsychologi-
cal and spiritual needs of the patient and their family. Most emphasized
the importance of tailoring care to the individual's needs following a
health assessment.

Demonstrating effective communication meant that, by achieving effective
interpersonal skills, better care could be achieved. Caring was the awareness of self-values, the ability to express oneself, sensitively perceiving
clients' thoughts and feelings and the ability to enhance patients' self-
concepts.

Providing a safe environment was considered very important as it supported
care in a situation where the nurses could provide safe support for their
patients. In addition to this, again, positive role-modelling from the senior nurses was seen as being extremely important in enhancing the
caring ethos amongst the care team.

What makes a 'good' nurse?

If one equates nurses and nursing with care, does it follow that an exploration of 'good' nursing gives a greater insight into care and caring? In
this respect it is, of course, of vital importance to understand and attempt
to measure patients' views of the above questions; they, after all, are on the
receiving end of what we do! In achieving this insight into what our
patients rate as good care, it is helpful to have some clear understanding of
the ways that patients experience illness, and how they perceive the ways
they believe nurses can help them to come to terms with or overcome illness. As Williams (1998) points out, while the theoretical meaning and
significance of caring are being discussed within the nursing profession,
the significance of nurse caring to patients is personal and not theoretical.

Riemen (1986) recounts this sad description of a qualified nurse by a
student nurse. 'She is always in a hurry; she didn't have time to talk, or,
even if she had time, she didn't really seem to want to talk. Her body language let me know she wasn't interested in what I had to say. All she was
here to do was to perform her duty and go home. She stood at a distance.
She didn't even come close.' Riemen then asked patients what they saw
non-caring behaviour to be. She found that they tallied with the student's
perceptions in several ways.

Bad nurses appeared to be efficient and in a hurry
Specific examples include:

- always in a hurry
- no time to talk
- super-efficient attitude

Bad nurses appeared to be just doing a job
Specific examples include:
- there to perform duties and then go home
- nothing seemed to bother the nurse – it was just a job

Bad nurses appeared to be rough and belittle their patients
Specific examples include:
- made me feel like a little kid
- she just wasn't soft
- talked loud and acted like I'd lost my marbles

Bad nurses did not respond
Specific examples include:
- didn't pay any attention
- she would not come back to help
- too busy talking to the other nurses to talk to me

Bad nurses appeared to treat patients as objects
Specific examples include:
- bathed me as though she was doing a dog
- looked at equipment and not at me

Riemen's very disturbing findings highlighted the way that, sometimes, nurses did not seem to make effective contact with the patients. Patients, it seems from this study, want nurses to spend time with them and (not surprisingly) to treat them with respect and dignity. Good nurses do make time for the patients. However, with the current shortfall of nurses and the increased activity that is apparent in British healthcare, it is of concern that time is less and less available for meaningful quality contact between patients and nurses.

Taylor (1993) also undertook research into what it was that made nurses most effective in the eyes of patients. Patients stated that it was not the most efficient or necessarily the most knowledgeable nurse who they viewed as being the best. Instead, it was the nurse who interacted with them in the most ordinary ways. The word 'ordinary' was interpreted as meaning a simple and uncomplicated openness between nurse and patient. Arguably, some of the most effective and pleasurable moments achieved when nursing patients are those where a rapport is achieved with the patient and their family that is open and frank. When nurses actually achieve this open relationship with patients and their family or loved ones they can then nurse on a totally different plane both in a physical and psychological way. It is then that nurses can be most effective.

Poole and Rowat, in their 1994 study, examined elderly home-care clients' perceptions of caring behaviours of nurses within the context of the nursing relationship. Their findings mirrored other research into this question in as much as it was the nurses' personal/psychological attributes that were considered as being of prime importance to the patient.

Good attributes were good mood, understanding, genuineness, patience and respect. It was, of course, important to patients that nurses were able to provide physical and organizational aspects of care but to a significantly lesser extent than the psychosocial aspects. This may be, at least in part, due to the nature of the relationship between nurses and patients, which is not as focused upon physical care as might be the case in the hospital, hospice or care-home setting.

One particularly interesting aspect of the study highlights the potential differences that gender may influence in perceptions of care. The researchers in their conclusion propose that male patients seemed to value technical performance and physical care over more affective nursing behaviours. Another explanation may lie in the feeling of discomfort in male patients in admitting that affective factors are important to their caring experience. This may be in part due to a macho view of care by some men in the West.

Conclusion

This chapter reveals some highly important insights into the way that nurses and patients perceive not just what care might be to them but also what they perceive their role is in relation to the actual caring process might be for the patient. The studies tend to show that nurses value most highly the interpersonal aspects of the caring relationship. It is the so-called 'touchy feely' parts of nursing that they believe to be most important to the patient. It is certainly true to say that patients also value these humanistic aspects of care, but some of the studies do show an important mismatch or difference in the perceptions of patients and nurses.

As stated above, the most highly valued aspect of care for the nurse is creating a strong relationship with the patient, whereas the patient sometimes also values a high level of competency and skill in the nurse. In reality, of course, the patient is unlikely to say that they are not concerned with the relationship between them and the nurse. They would want both aspects of care, for without the ability to comfort and create a strong bond with the patient and their family, even the most skilled and competent nurse could not deliver their care properly.

The studies also show that perceptions of care and caring are in fact extremely context-dependent. Those who are very acutely ill are perhaps more focused on tasks and effective treatments; they, for instance, want the nurse to provide the right drug in the right dose at the right time. The patient who is terminally ill, who has symptomatic relief or in long-term care is arguably not so worried about physical, task-based care but will be wanting a close and meaningful relationship so they can share their fears, hopes and expectations with a trusted care partner. Indeed, the former acutely ill patient, when their condition has stabilized, will perhaps require and value a very different set of skills to be exhibited by the nurse. Perhaps the challenge of nursing is to be sensitive to the dynamic needs of all patients and blend the essential nurse caring skills, so that care can be given at exactly the right time with the right emphasis and in the right way.

CHAPTER FOUR

Can we teach care to student nurses?

Introduction

Over recent years, the number of papers considering education for caring, and research papers exploring student attitudes and understanding of caring, has steadily and significantly increased. The issues surrounding education for caring have gradually taken greater prominence alongside the general trend of increasing literature on care and caring. Nursing in conjunction with healthcare in general is definitely becoming more technically demanding, with nurses in all areas, not just critical-care units, using more and more pieces of highly complex equipment and gadgetry to care for their patients. Coupled with this is the ever-increasing throughput of patients and their growing levels of dependency. With this in mind, it is important that the education of 'care' as a subject needs to keep pace with the greater-than-ever technical aspects of the curriculum. This is as true for qualified nurses as it is for students.

Students' views of care education

Nurses seem to have a strong desire or need to care, and see care as something that can be enhanced or developed by education. As Hughes (1995) points out, the future nurse needs to focus on caring for the individual patient and not necessarily on becoming a technological wizard who assesses wires, tubes and machines. Nurses do, of course, need to be technologically highly skilled. Technology cannot be ignored: it is here, and can and does help us look after our patients. However, it is certainly true that the patient needs nurses to humanize and soften the technical aspects of medical treatment and care.

Cohen (1993) believes that nurse education must be tuned to the values of caring and reflect the focus upon human care that stresses the holistic nature of people. This is so true, but let us explore further the emerging picture of what is happening in nursing education. Chipman (1991) carried out a qualitative study to help clarify the meaning and value of caring in nursing practice as perceived by 26 second-year nursing students. The students were asked to describe critical incidents in which they observed nursing behaviours conducted in caring and non-caring ways. Interestingly, none of the respondents talked about or wrote about technical competence as 'caring nurse' behaviour; however, this may be due to the relative lack of experience in the second-year students or the way that the question was asked. All of the nursing behaviours referred to were described in purely humanistic terms. When categorized, these behaviours feed into these overall themes:

- giving of self
- meeting patients' needs in a timely fashion
- providing comfort measures for patients and their families

Giving of self: in the eyes of the students this was exemplified by behaviours such as taking extra time with the patient or even spending off-duty time with the patient.

Meeting patients' needs: to the students this meant providing the patient with pain relief, attention, self-esteem, and meeting or helping to meet their religious requirements. Again, interestingly, none of the respondents referred to meeting the patients' most basic needs (food, fluid and elimination) as caring behaviours.

Providing comfort: the student respondents considered this factor as highly important. Behaviours such as easing psychological discomfort, grief, fear, anxiety and depression were seen as central to caring. This was also true in the case of the provision of a calming, soothing environment. The respondents also described several non-caring behaviours, such as not immediately helping patients, not providing privacy, disregarding patients' dignity and not using tact when dealing with patients and/or their families.

Nurse educators' perceptions of care

A better understanding of nurse educators' perceptions of caring is clearly important to providing a full picture of education for care. Komorita et al. (1991) surveyed 110 members of the education faculty to assess their views on the most- and least-caring behaviours. The ten highest scores were as follows:

- listens to patients
- allows patients to express feelings about their illnesses
- realizes patients knows themselves the best and includes them in their own care
- touches patients when they need comforting
- is perceptive of patients' needs and provides care accordingly
- gets to know patients as individuals
- talks to patients
- teaches patients self-care if possible
- encourages questions
- tells patients what is important to know about their illness

The teachers did not seem to value very highly the physical aspect of care or, indeed, the competency of these aspects of care. The ten least-caring behaviours perceived by them were:

- is calm
- checks the best time to talk with patients about condition
- gives treatments and medications on time
- knows when to call the doctor
- volunteers to do 'little things' for patients
- realizes that nights are the most difficult times for patients
- is well organized
- is cheerful
- suggests questions for patients to ask the doctor
- is professional in appearance

Perhaps what we can see here is an important split between students' and teachers' views of what caring behaviours might be. In the United Kingdom, teachers of nursing are drawn almost exclusively from the ranks of nurses, all with widely varying amounts of current practice with patients. This variation can range from no real current nursing input to an equal balance between teaching and practice, as with some lecturer practitioners. It is fair to say that there is present in nurse educators a varying level of remoteness from practice. So, if one considers the education and transmission of caring attitudes to students, is it relevant to examine how nurse educators experience caring in their work situations, namely in the schools, colleges and universities where nurses are educated?

Grigsby and Megel (1995) studied the attitudes of seven nurse educators to understand better how caring is carried out in the school of nursing. Two emerging themes became evident:

- caring is connection
- caring is a pattern of establishing and maintaining relationships

Caring is connection: teachers overwhelmingly described connection with students as being vital to the relationship. They spoke of the importance of understanding and sharing the students' problems both at home and in work. They wanted to connect with their students and stated that to enjoy teaching they needed to feel a link not just with the student but also with fellow faculty members. Non-caring behaviours were associated with the prevention of that connection, for example denigrating students or not recognizing their uniqueness. Teachers felt uncared for at times by their colleagues and managers. This they felt led to feelings of anger, uncertainty and powerlessness.

Caring is a pattern of establishing and maintaining relationships: the teachers felt motivated to develop relationships when peers and managers cared for and about them. They used different teaching methods to enhance their connection with the students. Another positive tool identified by the educator that enhanced the ability to teach caring was to help students care for their patients in the clinical area. Humour, listening, sharing ideas and sharing observations of both negative and positive caring behaviours were all seen as ways of getting to know better another faculty member, student or patient as a person. When teachers did not feel valued, they described either withdrawing from colleagues or secretly maintaining connections with those who they knew cared about them. The report concluded that nurse educators must explore how to promote caring experiences in the schools of nursing to help establish true communities of caring. Unfortunately, it is my experience that in some schools of nursing, student nurses are treated as though they are children and at times with little or no regard for their needs.

The students' perceptions of caring behaviour in education

Dillon and Stines (1996) undertook a study of 81 student nurses; they asked the students to respond to the following request: 'Describe in your own words one incident you have had with a faculty member whom you felt was caring.' The findings supported the view that it was important that the teacher established a climate in which caring is nurtured and valued. The students saw respect from the teacher as a critical prerequisite for an atmosphere of caring. Sharing and giving of oneself was also important: the giving of time to the student was highly valued – as was remembering the little things and listening. It was believed that students who were educated in this humanistic environment had a greater potential to carry this attitude to their practice.

In a similar study by Hanson and Smith (1996), 28 students were surveyed to better understand caring and not-so-caring interactions. The views expressed in this were very similar to those rehearsed in Dillon and Stines' study. Descriptions of the not-so-caring behaviours were expressed in ways such as 'the teacher had no time for me', 'was unavailable', 'condescending', 'dismissive' and 'disrespectful of students'. These types of interactions and behaviours caused students to feel rejected, cheated, powerless and discouraged.

It is clearly plausible to suggest that if one can foster an environment where teachers and students feel valued and motivated it is likely that a humanistic approach to nursing may be sown which will carry through into practice. In addition to this it must be true that effective teaching and learning can be far better achieved in a positive atmosphere.

Teaching care

What is the actual process of teaching care to student nurses? Simonson (1996) asks how teachers help students understand caring and how they foster and promote caring nursing behaviours in students. To this I would add the question: 'Is the teaching or transmission of genuine care possible, especially when one accepts the difficulty of the concept of care?' Eriksson (1992) states that nurses had acquired this knowledge and tendency to care by observing and working alongside their mothers in a family setting. This raises further the issue of how much influence nurse educators have in teaching care to students.

Bassett (1994a) outlines the often powerful effect and importance that secondary socialization plays in the journey the student nurse makes, pointing out that the education and training that the student nurse receives is highly influential in any future role undertaken and in the way nurses practise their care. Hughes (1995), an educator of nurses, reinforces this; she underlines the effect that the education process can have on caring attitudes in new nurses. Gratification of human need, development of a helping relationship and instillation of the ability to provide patients with faith and hope were all aspects that she felt could be taught or transmitted to nurses. Reinforcing this sentiment, Berman (1988) states that for most professions it is important to transmit the theory and knowledge to its students but in nursing it is crucial. To this I would also add the ethical and moral underpinnings of unique care. This care is what Eyles (1995) terms 'informed' care, that is, care underpinned by technical skill, and education supported by a philosophical basis. Simonson (1996) used phenomenology to better understand the processes teachers used to convey that caring is the essence of nursing, which students should learn. She wanted to describe what was occurring from the perspective of the participants. Six teachers were interviewed and asked to talk about the integration of caring in the teaching. Twelve students were also included in the research, and they were asked about the importance of knowledge of values of care, and how they were learning these values. Using Watson's (1979) model of her theory of human care (see Chapter Two's section 'Care: some points of view') as a means of organizing the research findings, the following linking factors were identified:

The formation of a humanistic-altruistic system of values: the teachers said things like: 'I hope the long-term message of my teaching is that I care about what happens to people.' Sentiments also included the importance of valuing people as individuals, as people with real and valuable feelings. Students echoed these views, saying that it was important to respect patients' values and care for them as individuals despite sometimes being from different cultures.

The cultivation of sensitivity to one's self and to others: teachers here placed great value on openness between them and their colleagues; they felt that this served as a good role model to the students. They talked about self-awareness as being important and not imposing their views and standards on others. Students made reference to the importance of having compassion, sensitivity and empathy for patients. One student felt that her teacher helped her to look at herself more effectively, increasing her self-awareness.

The promotion of interpersonal teaching/learning: teachers spoke of adapting students' individual learning to reflect their own individual culture, that is, some students were from Native American or Hispanic cultural backgrounds. Other students found it extremely useful when teachers referred to their own previous nursing experiences; this helped them relate caring to actual practice. Good caring teachers were those who showed genuine concern and care for the student. Teachers were not just seen as sources of information but as emotional and personal supporters as well.

The provision for a supportive, protective and/or corrective mental, physical, sociocultural and spiritual environment: teachers stated that it was important to provide for the patient a situation that did not question their own decision or belief system. It was not seen as the nurses' role to make decisions for the patient but to provide support while the patient made that decision. Students believed that the role of the nurse was to care for the whole family group; every person needed individual help to get through difficult situations. Meeting the patients' or their families' needs (be they spiritual, emotional or physical) was seen as vital.

The students seemed to find the teaching staff highly influential in the way they devised teaching strategies to underpin the caring aspects of nursing. The teachers also created a supportive, open and humanistic environment that again supported caring tendencies in the students.

Higgins (1996) believes that caring outcomes in practice depend on a caring teaching/learning process. She implemented a project aimed at underlining the subject of caring as a therapeutic entity in nursing practice. The goals of the project were to enable students to:

- encourage dialogue and share their stories, and to experience themselves as cared for
- manifest professional caring by implementing knowledge and intentional actions for the ultimate good of the patient

The programme of teaching devised a weekly meeting of the students – the purpose was to encourage them to support one another. Stories that persuaded them to become nurses were exchanged, and many powerful accounts of caring reasons were voiced. As the course continued, the aim of increasing self-esteem became prominent, and the use of reflective diaries and strong positive group support helped students to foster caring attitudes. In addition to this, the course was also aimed at providing professional insights into how nurses can enhance the caring ethos in the clinical area. The students met patients to understand their experiences, and this helped them to generally feel more at ease as a new nurse in practice. This approach of creating caring groups can be seen as a potentially sensitive and supportive introduction to nursing practice for the new student; early exposure to the harsh realities of nursing can at times be traumatic and even damaging to the new nurse.

Grams et al. (1997) wanted to understand better the effects of creating caring groups as a strategy to learn caring. Twenty-five students were included in the study and they expressed feelings that were clustered into three patterns or themes:

Creating the caring community: following the setting of rules, the group established trust and began to see the faculty as part of the group. The teachers were seen as facilitators of the processes in the group.

Experiencing the reciprocity of caring: terms like 'sharing care experiences', 'experiencing the reciprocity of caring', 'bonding' and 'self-disclosure' were used to describe the group's work. They became a place of support, encouragement and commitment to helping other students get through.

Being transformed: participants spoke of being transformed as a result of the experience. They felt they were able to see others in a holistic way, self-understanding was boosted and they felt they were better placed to care for others personally and professionally.

The findings concluded that nurses can learn care from teachers if trust and commitment are present. The researchers felt encouraged that ex-participants were able to create climates of care following graduation.

Students from different cultures

Many new nurses in the UK are recruited from other countries, and this trend is increasing. Kosowski et al. (1997) carried out research into the effects of caring groups in education, in this case with students from different countries, including the US, Nigeria, India, China and Chile. The research findings were of great interest, as the participants freely discussed the issues of being from different countries and cultures. The processes of the group were similar to Grams et al. (1997), and the expressed views of the group were also similar. Mutual support and an increase in self-awareness and understanding were highly valued. The international group also spoke of being changed in certain ways by the group. They identified new ways of being people and nurses. They described feeling better able to spend more focused time with their patients. The students in this study described a very positive outcome to their participation in the care groups, which they would take back with them to implement in their own countries' health systems.

Wilkes and Wallis (1998) carried out a study to describe the construct of caring as experienced by Australian students. Questionnaires and interviews were used, and the sampled students were selected from each of the three years of the course. The researchers wanted to understand better how students' views of caring altered over three years of nurse education. The students over the three years are taught, and experience, ways of actualizing the caring attitudes that they bring with them to nursing, through relationships within a nursing context. The researchers, through analysing the data, noticed a theory of student perceptions of caring begin to emerge (Figure 4.1).

Major themes	Definition
compassion	love and friendship, being concerned for another
communication	verbal, non-verbal and physical contact
concern	the students used this word
competence	the ability to use cognitive, affective and psychomotor skills
commitment	doing things they did not want to do
confidence	being able to do things without doubting oneself
conscience	taking account of their actions
courage	standing up for the patient

Figure 4.1 Wilkes and Wallis' 1998 model of students' experience of caring.

This model of care seems to show a high level of understanding of the caring factors involved in professional nursing. The research stops short of claiming that caring attitudes can be taught. What it does indicate though is that new students bring with them compassion and other caring attributes that can be focused and enhanced by both education and practical experience.

The experience that students receive in the clinical setting is also considered by many as being highly influential in the way they learn to care. Wong and Lee (2000) point out that a positive practice environment can enhance the professional development of the student nurse and can in fact influence decisions of student nurses to stay in or leave nursing. Close collaboration is needed between education and practice to ensure that there is a close relationship between the two areas. Good education received in the classroom can be enhanced by the student's clinical experience just as easily as it can be damaged. In another study, Tennant (1999) explored the perceptions of nine new recruits to nursing. The majority of the students had a perception of nursing and caring as very much one of helping others; this seemed to be a very practically based perception: 'Doing things for the patient.' This perhaps indicates a somewhat naive view of nursing possessed by the students. Providing comfort was also seen as important, and there was a strong feeling that caring as a nurse necessitated a strong bond being formed between nurse and patient.

Nurturing was another emergent category; one of the nurse's roles was seen as that of educator and health promoter. Encouraging the patient to take a more active role in their treatment was also considered important, even if that involved the patient's participation up to and until their death. Helping the patient get better (healing) was part of the nurses' perception of caring as a nurse. The doctor–nurse relationship was seen as a team effort aimed at working towards successful treatment. Finally, the respondents identified that unpaid and untrained people undertake a great deal of nursing. They saw care as not exclusive to nurses but felt that nurses have a great deal to offer in terms of specialist skills and knowledge. The concept of correct conduct and professionalism was also identified in the research.

As mentioned earlier, the perceptions of the students were clearly in some ways immature; however, certain aspects of the research were surprisingly insightful. For instance, the issues surrounding the increasing need for stronger levels of autonomy and accountability in modern nursing practice were identified, and also how the increase in other caring bodies and alternative or complementary medical practitioners means nurses are not the only people who can care for patients.

Conclusion

All who have an interest in nursing will no doubt have a view on the best ways to educate nurses to ensure that their practice is underpinned by sound principles of caring theory. It is clearly extremely valuable to understand the attitudes and beliefs of student nurses towards their future role as carers. We all have a great opportunity to ensure that the professional nurses of the future – who will, after all, be looking after us – have the best start. The debate over the place for nurse education in the UK (university, college or hospital) is still being carried out some five or six years after it has actually moved into higher education (HE). As Fletcher (1997) points out, the move into HE offers an unprecedented opportunity for nursing to realize fully its professional aspirations to be a caring profession. Van der Wal (1999) believes that nursing students' main quest is to attribute meaning to their working life through caring for patients. This being true, the onus must surely therefore be on teachers of nursing to plan curricula and teaching methods that support the needs of students and ultimately, of course, those of the patients.

CHAPTER FIVE

Making a connection

Introduction

So at last we have reached the chapters that allow us to read and try to understand what the nurses themselves say, think and feel about what they do. There can be little doubt that creating a relationship between nurses and patients is essential for effective nursing care to take place. Making a connection is the first theme that will be examined in relation to the expressed sentiments of the nurses. The expressed feelings, attitudes and beliefs describe ways of caring that epitomize the perceived closeness that is required by the nurse to care for the patient. In their narratives, they mentioned more than just one theme; it is inevitable in this kind of interview that there is a crossover of themes. In describing their expressed views and beliefs throughout the following chapters, these allied expressions are not always removed from the whole transcribed section. Some of the extracts illustrate more than one theme, and this will be noted in the discussion of the extract. However, extracts have been grouped according to the main theme they illustrate. This chapter is really about nurses' communication with their patients.

Aspects of making a connection

Anne, who works half her time in the operating theatre, stated in her interview that it was important to her to be there for the patient. Despite the obvious issues with many of her patients being unconscious for a lot of the time while in her care, Anne considered patient connection as being important. She explained it in this way:

> **Chris**: Theatres are not the place that you have as much patient contact as other areas.

Anne: Yes, I'd have to agree with you on that one because obviously the majority of the time the patient is actually asleep, but I think it depends on what you mean by 'patient contact'. I perceive that the care that is given – although the patient might not be awake the same care is given – and that you give the care to the patient throughout the peri-operative period, some of which will be given to the patient in the reception area when the patient is awake, which is seen as high-care hands-on patient areas – as is recovery, where the patient is awake again after the surgery. The in-between times don't seem to be very high-patient-contact time, but personally I think that is the main time that the patient does need the care that is provided by the nursing staff, because the patient is in a very vulnerable position.

Anne seems to understand her responsibility very clearly towards her patients. In the operating theatre it seems at times that there is a clearly defined process at play; it is somewhat like a factory or assembly plant, with patients being the product moving through the process. The theatre itself is like a clean environment where computer chips are assembled. There is little or no sign of a human softening of the environment, which is altogether harsh and white. It could be easy for the nurse to forget the patient and become preoccupied with the process. Despite the environment in theatre, Anne sees care of the patient as the central part of her work in the operating theatre.

Chris: Of all the factors in your job, what is the most important to you?

Anne: I think it's got to be being there for the patient. I think if anybody who's in professions allied to nursing says anything other than the patient care and making sure that we care for them to the best of our ability, which is difficult these days, they are wrong. I have had experience of being a patient myself, and it is very, very important to both the patient and the relatives that they know that the nurses are looking after them.

As Anne notes above, actual experience of being in hospital or having relatives in hospital helps nurses understand the issues of being cared for.

One might argue that nurses sometimes have allowed the medical model, with its associated technology, to dominate their practice at the expense of patient care; Anne has chosen to place her patient at the centre of her care. Theatre, in common with many other high-technology areas, can be described as a place where nurses are involved in very highly intensive processes.

Jill also works in theatres; in her interview she felt that the emotional issues were of real importance to her care. Tournier (1985) believes we are bound up with a technological civilization; this can be readily transferred to healthcare. Tournier points out that we have constructed a world of hardness with things taking precedence over the person. The expressed views of Jill illustrate the way in which she seems to work against the hardness of things in her practice.

> **Chris**: What would be the most important part of being a nurse?
>
> **Jill**: It's difficult to split it because you've got to give the physical care: make sure that they are physically safe, that the patients are safe. But it's the caring aspect, looking after the emotional side of it.

There is clearly a need, according to Jill, to invest an emotional element into her caregiving. Geekie and Grieve (1997) point out that nurses need to find ways to help the patient through potentially frightening experiences by helping patients see nurses in theatre as people who are human and who are ready to spend time with their patients. They speak of meeting patients prior to surgery in pre-operative visiting clinics; this is a way that they see they can help overcome the fear of surgery.

Lynn works in day surgery. This type of care is very rapid in its turnover; there is very little time to spend with the patient prior to theatre.

> **Chris**: Can you tell me a bit about where you work and your role?
>
> **Lynn**: I work on day surgery as a senior staff nurse, and I have face-to-face contact with patients, a very high turnover of patients, and we have a caseload of between three to five patients in a morning and the same in the afternoon. We do keep patients in all day, and that gives us a whole day to get to know them, but basically it's very fast turnover and not much time to make any sort of relationship with anybody, although we do try ... well, I try. So you've got to be very skilled at being able to anticipate their needs and to support them and know what it is they're worried about very quickly, because sometimes you've only got an hour before they're off to theatre.

Here we can see that the nature of day surgery is perhaps different from many wards in hospital in that it has a very rapid patient turnover; however, it can be argued that nursing time in almost all areas of practice is becoming squeezed, with increased throughput of patients and shortened stays in hospital. In the light of this reduced time, it is a real challenge to develop a relationship with the patient in such a comparatively short time.

Tuning in

The ability to develop a quick relationship with the patient is not necessarily inbuilt in all nurses; there is a process that nurses pass through that enables this ability to 'tune in' to the patient in a rapid manner. Benner (1984) describes the process leading from novice to expert. It is characterized by the movement from novice, where rule-based practice is used, through to expert carer, where the nurse no longer relies on the analytical principle. Instead the nurse develops an intuitive grasp of each situation, much like Lynn with her ability to tune in. Lynn describes her ability to identify patients who are perhaps not coping well or are worried about their operation. She points out ways in which she picks up non-verbal cues and uses these as prompts for her care. Lynn is an expert nurse; she has a large amount of experience caring for patients. She demonstrates in her narrative an intuitive grasp of the situation. Lynn seems to work from a deep understanding of the total situation. There is a possibility that nurses may find this frustrating and lead to their not enjoying their time in this area. I wondered how Lynn felt this factor affected her ability to care.

Chris: Do you find that [rapid turnover] frustrating?

Lynn: Well, I did at first because you just don't feel like you are preparing people and at the moment we've not really got any pre-admission clinics where we can actually prepare people, but in fact you do become skilled at it and tune in more or less straight away. If you meet somebody and you can see that they are relaxed and you can get a picture of what they are worried about, then you can tune in and you do get skilled. It's easy to pick out if people have problems. If they come in and you sense that there is something wrong either because they are not communicating, they won't look at you or they've got their relatives very close by and you can actually pick up [on that], and that becomes a skill. It's through dealing with a lot of people coming in that are vulnerable and anxious. There is no way that you can be prepared for that, because it's not like any other ward. Even outpatients is different again because you are not really in a contact ... it's a very short period of time.

Here Lynn identifies the difficulties of working in such a short period of time with her patients, and she feels has developed ways of quickly identifying the needs of her patients. She felt able to tune in to their needs. Her early frustration seemed to reduce as she became more attuned to her patients' specific care needs in day surgery. Lynn is showing a high level of functioning here; she is working through and around problems to provide a high level of care for her patients.

Chris: What attributes are essential to a nurse?

Lynn: One of them has to be understanding the patient. You can't go into a life-long history, but, if you can, in day surgery, we only have a few minutes to find out about people. If you can find out and be understanding of the way that they are feeling and why they are coming in and what they are worried about etc. I don't know what the word is. It's not really empathy; it's some sort of understanding of what they may be feeling. I suppose it's sympathy really, but, if you can do that, it gives you a better base on which to communicate back to them and what their needs are. It's about assessing people so you know where they're coming from, you know where their worries are and you know where to focus.

'Empathy' is a word that is frequently used by nurses to describe a way of caring for their patients. However, despite its common usage, empathy remains, to me, an elusive concept. One person's lived experience is unique; arguably it cannot be truly understood by another. It can only ever be a partial understanding. What is required in empathy is a sufficient projection of self into the private world of the other, to be able (at least partially) to understand effectively what the experience means for them. Kunyk and Olson (2001) describe empathy as a professional state or set of skills composed primarily of behavioural and cognitive components that are used to convey understanding of the patient's realities back to them. Lynn seems to be using it in this sense to enhance her caring.

In addition to the use of professional empathy in care, it may be that a sign of an effective nurse is the ability to cut to the chase, as it were, and rapidly assess the patient and help them cope with their illness or operation (Benner 1984).

> **Chris**: How might you define 'caring'?
>
> **Lynn**: To sort of tune in. What I'm trying to say is that you might do something out of your own needs to care for somebody without actually defining what they want. So maybe it's a reciprocal understanding that you are not doing things for somebody else because you need to care for them or it might be that you do something or care about somebody else in a way that you want to be cared for, but in fact it's not about knowing what other people want and then responding to that. I don't think I have a definition, but maybe you can draw something from that! The main point I'm trying to say is that caring is not something that you feel that you need to do and you can say, 'I've done that for that person, that means I'm caring for them,' because it may be that that person doesn't want that doing. I think it all revolves around communication and interaction.

For some nurses humour was seen as an important way to establish and maintain a caring connection with their patients.

Humour

May was a very experienced ear, nose and throat (ENT) sister. She was about to leave nursing shortly after the interview with me. She was disillusioned with nursing and wanted to leave some years before she would have normally retired.

> **Chris**: What kind of nurses do you think are the best kind of nurses?
>
> **May**: The best kind of nurse? I want them to have a good brain. They need it in this job. They have to apply the knowledge they have learnt. I like them to

have a sense of humour; a sense of humour gets us over everything. To be able to stand back and have a good laugh at yourself; it does help, you know?

Humour in nursing is seen by some nurses to be important to them. It seems to be a way to overcome stressful or emotionally demanding situations and also a way to help the patient feel better cared for.

Chris: Can I ask you for any situations that you can recall from your nursing career that epitomize the way you got your care across to the patient and how they felt about it?

May: There are so many that it's difficult to pick one out. There was just one [which] raised tears in so many people's eyes, and I sat and laughed and laughed and laughed. There was a gentleman, again major surgery; he'd got carcinoma. He'd had half his tongue removed, but he would be able to eat again pretty normally. He'd had half his mandible removed, resection of the floor of his mouth, and he'd had a tracheotomy in just really for elective purposes just for the surgery. He did develop swallowing difficulties after, and they decided to keep the tracheotomy tube in. Now somewhere along the line this man had understood that this tube would perhaps be in for months and months and months, and his wife had recently left him, and he had married a younger lady, and I changed his tracheotomy tube for one that had a speaking valve in it, and he found all this very traumatic. He was very upset. He didn't like this tube being changed a bit, and his eyes were flashing at me as if to say, 'What more are you going to put me through?' I popped in and said, 'When your wife comes, you'll be able to say "I love you"; won't you practise it?' He went, 'I love you', and tears were pouring down his face, and all the other nurses started crying with him, and I just sat there with him and laughed and laughed and laughed and laughed! That part to me is just caring and loving, knowing the right thing to say because I knew he cared very much, and I felt that he was worried that because he had recently been married and he was older than his wife that she wouldn't be able to cope with the altered way he looked, and I felt that he needed some kind of reassurance. They fell into one another's arms ... I pulled the curtains round, and we let them get on with it.

May, in her interesting and amusing description of the use of humour in nursing, is describing the ability to use humour to defuse painful or embarrassing situations. It can help the nurse to cheer up the patient, to reduce stress in both patient and nurse. Healy (2000) suggests that the use of humour in nursing can be effective in this stress reduction and found that humour acted as a buffer on the worst effects of negative mood states. Asrdt-Kurki and Isola (2001), in their study on the use of humour between nurses and their patients, also found that nurses use humour for a variety of reasons with their patients. The study showed that humour between nurses and patients enabled both parties to cope with the different care routines, unpleasant procedures and with embarrassing situations, and I think the example above illustrates this well. It should be pointed out that the use of humour could be dangerous in certain situations, as a nurse may offend a patient or their family by the use of misplaced or hurtful humour. May seemed to have got it right in this situation.

Getting involved

Mike is a lecturer who is skilled and experienced in cancer-care nursing. He feels that to care fully one needs to be involved.

Chris: What part of your caring role did you find most interesting?

Mike: Patient relationships. I was really interested in how the patient responded to a diagnosis of cancer and how that affected them, and so it was about communicating. I really enjoyed talking to them, communicating with the patients, finding out what made them tick and how diagnosis of cancer affected that.

Rittman et al. (1997) state that knowing the patient (in this case the cancer patient) is vital to the care of that patient. In addition to understanding the ways that the patient reacts to their illness diagnosis, it is considered as essential to relate knowledge of the patient to the illness trajectory. In Rittman et al.'s study, the nurses described developing a 'special bond' with patients as an important ingredient when they engage in 'death work' with patients.

Chris: Would you consider yourself to be a caring person?

Mike: I would hope so. Yes, I think that's one of the things about oncology is the fact that the carer is very much psychologically orientated and very much orientated to caring. Whereas in some other areas it's very much task-orientated, but within oncology, caring for the psychosocial needs of the patient is very important, and therefore that is a great part of caring for somebody.

Chris: What do you consider to be the most important part of your job in cancer care?

Mike: Actually talking to the patient and communicating with them. Because without that you can't get to know what the patient is thinking, how they are going to respond to specific situations, and I think you need to have that knowledge to provide competent care. You can have the skills, but it's how you deliver those skills to the patient, and therefore you need to be able to talk to and communicate with them to find all those things out.

Mike is describing expert caring practice (Benner 1984); his belief is that becoming involved with his patients and their family is key to high-quality caring. As Gay (1999) points out, getting involved with patients requires attentive listening; this is a key prerequisite to caring. Attentive listening allows patients and family members to verbalize their fears and concerns, and nurses to elicit any expectations or, indeed, misconceptions. Nurses who are skilful listeners use verbal and non-verbal behaviours, for example facial expressions, eye contact, body movements, distance, silence, touch and voice intonations. In short, how nurses interact with patients can be as therapeutic as the physical care they provide.

In terms of technology, intensive-care nursing is perhaps at the other end of the caring spectrum. Steve is a senior staff nurse in intensive care but also spends approximately half his time teaching students in the classroom. Intensive-care nursing is a highly specialized role with a great deal of one's time spent checking, maintaining and operating highly complex pieces of life-support equipment. In addition to this, the patients are usually unconscious or unable to communicate with nurses or relatives, owing to the nature of their illness or the invasive nature of their life-support systems.

One might wonder what type of nurse wants to work in this environment; it seems to almost be the antithesis of care. The patient is usually unable to speak or may be unconscious. Sometimes one has to rely on the patient's relatives to find out about the patient. The nurse also often spends long periods of time with the relatives and has to care for them as much as they do for the patients themselves. This is clearly reflected in Steve's expressed views.

> **Chris**: What do you find most satisfying about intensive care?
>
> **Steve**: The main thing is that I've got time to spend with patients that I'm looking after and their families, and my job is very patient-centred.
>
> **Chris**: What about the relatives? Usually, there are relatives present all the time. What about them? How do you relate to them?
>
> **Steve**: I'm a big believer in things being easier if you have lots of information about it and being aware what possibilities there are in the future and that kind of thing. So a lot of my practice is based on information-giving, making things meaningful for them and answering their questions. I try and put myself in their position as much as possible. That's some of the motivation for my relationship with them: building my relationship with them and giving them the care that I do with the family. There are obviously people that I don't like, but that often affects the relationship, and sometimes people come across as 'copers' and obviously they don't need as much intervention – as much information – as people that don't seem to be coping. That affects my relationship with them and what I actually do with them or say to them.

Steve is describing how he manages to balance high-technology nursing with his ideals of care – thus, as he sees it, overcoming the barriers that technology might bring to the development of a caring relationship.

Schoenhofer and Boykin (1998) believe that, when nurses enter a nursing situation, practising from a medical-science perspective, the focus of practice tends to be skewed to the 'problem of the part' and the nurses tend to prescribe other technological interventions to correct the problem. Steve here is describing the way he prescribes a non-technological approach; he finds time to connect with patients and their families to help them.

Mary is a sister on the post-anaesthetic care unit (PACU). She likes to get involved with her patients.

> **Chris**: So what is the most satisfying part?
>
> **Mary**: It's the patient contact side of things, and a nice thing that happens at my unit is our recovery staff, pre-op, visit the patients. The same nurse then tries to bring the patient up to theatre, take them into the anaesthetic room, stay with them until they are on the operating table, bring them into recovery, nurse them, take them back and hand over. So they really get attention, because I think that's lacking in other operating departments. Some people even get on patients' nerves, but we have looked after that patient right from the pre-operative visit. Sometimes we even get to know the families if they are there when we visit. Then we are taking other patients back to the ward and patients are waving to us.

Apart from nurses' believing that effective and incisive communication is an essential part of the caring process, it would appear that the achievement of this also provides nurses with a great deal of personal satisfaction in their role. Barker (2000) goes further in this direction; he speaks not just of satisfaction of the nurse in providing care but also of experiencing a kind of self-healing. So nursing and the provision of care may be more than altruism, more than financial benefits; it may, indeed, be nourishment for the nurses themselves. In considering these issues, we move into consequentialist, utilitarian and deontological areas of ethical debate, which, though interesting and perhaps fruitful, are beyond the scope of this study.

Sometimes two themes are closely interwoven, as seen with the themes 'getting involved' and 'being there'.

Getting involved and being there

Sue works in PACU also.

> **Chris**: What's your experience of caring for patients?
>
> **Sue**: Well, sometimes the ladies that are coming for evacuations – for the miscarriages – are really the majority of the time very, very upset. They just need to talk to somebody about it. There's that time to be able to do that basically. Sometimes the nurses on the ward haven't either got the time or they

don't feel comfortable so they can walk away, whereas when you are with your patient you stay with them. So you get an interaction.

McQueen's (1997) study is supported by Sue's feelings as expressed here. The nurses in McQueen's research often expressed some discomfort in caring for patients having terminations of pregnancy. The degree of empathy and engagement achieved was considered as important in being able to anticipate patients' needs, respond to subtle cues and to the extent to which nurses can care about, as opposed to care for, patients. It was seen very much as an area that can rigorously test emotional reserves in nurses.

I wanted to know more about Sue's views on the psychological aspects she particularly seemed to value in her caregiving.

Chris: So it's a listening thing?

Sue: Yes.

Chris: How long do you normally get with each patient?

Sue: It varies … we actually do our own escort service so that we've got that time as well; so you are probably talking 15–20 minutes before the operation and then afterwards, depending on the nature of the operation and how long they are in recovery for. Again, I think it's the talking, listening and things like that. Just being there for them to talk to somebody.

Sue saw her role very much as someone to listen or if necessary even to counsel her patients. Sue is clearly committed to participating in the human experience of loss. As Bertero (1999) indicates, nurses who practise caring must be able to take on the perspective of the patients and be touched by the situation of a fellow being. It is arguable that it is in caring that nurses and patients connect with each other, are fulfilled and experience growth.

Chris: So that's the most satisfying part, the counselling? How much of your nursing now in recovery is counselling and how much hands-on?

Sue: I think it can be as much as what you want it to be. You can either not do it or do it. So I quite like it; so I feel that I do quite a lot. So I would say probably as high as 40–60%, something like that.

Sue identified that some of her colleagues did not seem at ease with the intimate psychological aspects of care. She seemed to think that they did not perhaps care as much as they might for the patient.

Chris: So some of your colleagues, I take it, are much more happy to do the hands-on stuff and not get involved in counselling. How do you feel about that?

Sue: A bit sad really. But, like I said, sometimes that's their personality and they can't deal with it. I like dealing with awkward cases, mental illness I always tend to be picked to deal with, or offer to nurse them.

Sue indicates that, in her view, to care fully for her patients she needs to develop a close and intimate relationship with them. This to her seems to be the key to the caring therapeutic potential of her nursing. Williams (2001), in her research, using content analysis as a method, found that part of nursing intimacy as described by Sue included disclosure between patient and nurse. Vulnerability and the sharing of personal experiences seemed to underpin the caring role of the nurse. These factors also seem to be present in the following examples from community and psychiatric nursing.

Jackie is a practice nurse working in a general practitioner's surgery. Practice nursing is quite different from the role of the nurse working in a hospital setting. The practice nurse, it would appear, can achieve a closer relationship with the patient; there is more opportunity to build a long-term relationship with the patient.

Nurses in the primary-care sector, it can be argued, develop different ways of working from those of their hospital-based colleagues. Hugman et al. (1997) believe that nurses in primary healthcare tend to be concerned with individual clients' general circumstances and overall health status, as well as any immediate specific health problems. This would certainly seem to be the case with Jackie.

> **Chris**: Which part or parts of the job that you are in now have become particularly interesting?
>
> **Jackie**: Being involved in people's lives and their families and helping them make informed decisions about their health and even helping them come to terms with part of their health and bereavement. Even though I'm not qualified, I think it's more the support-counselling side that keeps my interest. I think a lot of it is giving psychological support ... I had a lady whose son had committed suicide and she hadn't told anybody else, and it's getting her in contact with someone who can help, and luckily we've got the psychiatric nurse coming in so I get quite a few people in contact with the psychiatric nurse, which I can do directly – even though officially it's through the GP. A lot of the job is just telling people they are on the right track and they're OK doing what they are doing. Like I say, it's listening out for what they need.

Cathy is a psychiatric nurse; she has also been a general nurse but decided to work in psychiatry. She saw 'being there' for her patients as an important part of caring for them.

> **Chris**: Do you have your own personal understanding of what it is to care for someone?
>
> **Cathy**: It's very difficult. It would have to be, for me, more than just doing things for somebody. It would have to be much more on an emotional level than that. A lot of times as a professional carer you have to care for people that you have strictly speaking no emotional connection with. In some way

you have to care on that level, to actually genuinely listen and hear what's really happening and to do things that are less tangible, to just say, 'Well, I'll sit here for a bit if that's helpful'; the softer things as well would be caring, I think.

It is unlikely that all students know how to make connections with patients; some may have pre-existing nursing experience or, owing to maturity, are better placed to make connections with patients. However, in common with other nursing practices, there are skills and techniques that need to be learned. This section describes the experiences of student nurses. It is notable that several of the themes mentioned by the more experienced nurses were echoed in some of the students' comments.

Learning to make a connection

I was impressed with the entire student group I spoke to about care and caring. Without doubt, they were all highly motivated and seemed generally excited by the training and experiences they were gaining. The students, even in their first year, were already picking up on the ways they might make effective connections. Empathy was seen as an important way of connecting with patients.

Alice is a second-year student nurse.

Chris: What are the essential things you need, to be a good nurse?

Alice: I think you need empathy; you need to have a love of people and want to care for people.

Chris: What do you think empathy is?

Alice: Understanding how people are feeling. How it's affecting them.

It may be difficult for Alice to be truly empathic towards her patients. She is a student nurse in her second year only. Without doubting her caring characteristics, it must be said that perhaps she is mirroring what she knows to be a valued concept in her teachers (the behavioural 'professional state' as described above by Kunyk and Olson 2001). Empathy is often spoken about in the classroom situation as being a prerequisite of 'good' nursing; it is a learned clinical skill (Alligood 1992). Alice is arguably learning what to say. It may be difficult for true empathy to be achieved for the reasons stated above, but, as Hare (1981) hints, even partial acquisition of these skills is useful, even desirable, in nursing care.

Chris: What makes someone a good nurse?

Alice: Good communication skills. Being able to listen and interpret, not just verbally but body language and ... another thing as well is intuition. I think you need to be intuitive because ... you do pick up on things that people don't say or that other people outside might see it. It's like fitting a jigsaw together; you might pick up on one thing and somebody else might mention it, and you think, well yeah, that fits. I feel that it's being at one with somebody. What happens to them happens to you as well.

Alice here is expressing a strong connectedness with her patients. She seems to be alluding to some of the sentiments expressed by the experienced nurses mentioned previously. She wanted to 'get involved' with and 'tune into' her patients.

Carl is a first-year student nurse. He seems to be impressed with the way that staff nurses tuned into their patients' needs.

Chris: What has impressed you in the way that nurses deal with their patients?

Carl: I suppose in the different areas that I've been exposed to I've been involved with, medical wards, surgical wards, paediatric wards, also a little bit of primary healthcare as well. I find that the key to it in my mind is the fact that the nurse, in his or her role, is able to perform the clinical duties that they have, but perhaps more noticeably. I think it is the way that they can relate to the individual and be able to identify that person's needs. And work with them in partnership. That's the thing I've been impressed with most; it's not just their sort of levels of competency as clinicians, but I personally feel that the key to it all as a practising clinician is the way you actually communicate with your clients. Then I think you're two-thirds of the way there, as it were.

Carl thought that it seemed to be the junior nurses who usually made the first connection with the patients:

Carl: My experience is that the ones that really are making a connection with the patients are the ones that, you know, are perhaps either newly qualified or who have a relatively lowly status in nursing terms. But, you know, who is first contact is the patient and not the administration or whatever.

Joan also reflected on situations in her training. She is a second-year student.

Chris: What aspects of behaviour do you consider as being caring?

Joan: I think it's the actual response between the individuals rather than what they actually do. I mean, you can just tell when you know a person is, you know, caring.

Chris: How do you tell?

Joan: I don't know. You just get this feeling. You might look at a distance and, I don't know, for some reason [from] their body language I think, oh yeah, this person's ... definitely feeling comfortable with the other person ... Person A is acting this way; person B is acting this way: hence there must be something quite good, something more deep going on.

Chris: Could you define 'care'?

Joan: I don't think there is ... a definition really. I mean, I can't think of one. I'll probably support, you know, the intuitive thing, what Benner suggested. But I wouldn't say, I don't know; you know as I said before I do think there's a lot to do with feeling and the way you respond to things – the way you interpret things, the way you do things. It's a real mixture of all sorts, really.

Jess, a second-year student, recalled a situation that had impressed her; she had witnessed a qualified nurse who had broken bad news to a relative:

> **Jess**: It was a young nurse who had to see recently bereaved family members, and one of them, the son of the person who had actually died, was unable to go in and be with his mum, and the nurse had dealt with all the aftercare of this patient [who] had actually died, and the relatives were in the waiting room, and we took the property through, and she actually showed that she had time to sit down and listen.

Jess echoed the more experienced nurses' views that 'being there' for the patients was important to the caring process; this too reflected some of the issues raised in William's (2001) study, particularly those relating to self-disclosure.

> **Jess**: She didn't enforce any of her opinions. She did introduce an experience, a personal experience, into the conversation. She didn't actually thrust it at them and said, well, if I were you and that sort of situation; she only offered the information as if to show that she understood the situation, and it was done really sensitively, and it did help him to decide that he would actually go and see his mum, and he did thank us after.

Williams (2001) points out that there are several different levels of disclosure. These range from the exchange of superficial information to the sharing of deeply held private secrets. What Jess describes is the way that the qualified nurse shared and disclosed with the worried son, thus enhancing the caring intervention. This is used in many instances in nursing, leading to a deeper kind of caring relationship in practice. Jess seems to value this and has begun to learn that this is a part of caring at a deeper level. Humour was seen as a way to make the patient feel more at ease by the qualified nurses, and this too was picked up on in the student interviews.

Learning to use humour

In common with some of her qualified colleagues, student nurse Paula also thought that humour was an important tool to use in caring.

Chris: What kinds of caring behaviour do you see from them [qualified colleagues]?

Paula: Well, I think that the caring behaviour that I admire is when the nurse I know can use their sense of humour or can give a patient a hug when they know that the patient needs a hug, or just comfort them by just being there. It depends – you can tell a good nurse from that.

Chris: You mentioned 'sense of humour'.

Paula: Caring is hard; sometimes by joking I think a nurse can bring out things that a patient isn't willing to come to terms with as well. Like joking: sometimes tongue-in-cheek, they can say something and the patient can realize that the nurse understands how they're feeling.

Therefore, it can be argued that even student nurses see the use of humour as an effective way of defusing awkward situations, allowing patients and nurses to become closer, thus enabling more effective care to be given.

Conclusion

Making a connection with the patient is important to nurses. They see it as a vital factor in the effectiveness of the relationship. This is also supported by the literature. Kovner (1989) states that the nurse–patient relationship is important for the achievement of a positive patient outcome. Recovery, comfort, health, behaviour and compliance are linked to the effectiveness or otherwise of the nurse–patient relationship (Lauer et al. 1982, Kincey and Kat 1984, Keane-McDermott et al. 1987).

In addition to this, nurses may not be able to even provide good nursing care to their patients without a satisfactory level of communication or contact. Petersson et al. (2000) state that if nurses depend solely on information given on admission, or on their own assumptions, they may be unable to meet the care needs of those patients. Holistic nursing practice can be seen as taking care a step further. Simpson (1999) takes Petersson et al.'s view a stage further; she points out that holistic nursing is not necessarily something that we do; it is more an attitude or a philosophy, or a way of being. Simpson sees a nurse's way of being as a critical contribution in the act of caring.

Humour was also seen as important to caring; humour may be a factor in the process of creating a togetherness or partnership with the patient (Williams 2001). It may also be one way to relieve stress in patients and nurses. McGhee (1998) writes that humour itself has certain positive effects on the immune system and has been shown to reduce pain in certain situations. Laughter may be the best medicine. However, it is unlikely that nurses instinctively induce humour in their patients to stabilize their

physical conditions. Instead, it is more likely a way to defuse embarrass-
ment and to promote a partnership with their patients, and also to have
fun while at work.

Many of the nurses interviewed in this present study do seem to place a
great value upon making a connection with patients, but, despite them
speaking eloquently and at some length about tuning in and communicating, it is still not entirely clear that nurses communicate as well as they may
think with their patients. Further research is needed to measure this. The
student co-researchers at times seemed to mirror the expressed sentiments
of the qualified nurses. This mirroring perhaps reflects the strong influence that the more experienced nurses had in transmitting to the students
the importance of involvement in the caring process. This role-modelling
tendency was evident throughout the study in the other themes.

CHAPTER SIX

Encouraging autonomy

Introduction

The issues of encouragement of patient autonomy and the empowerment of patients seem to be important to the nurses in this study. Their importance is reflected by some of the published literature measuring patients' attitudes towards nursing care. Hankela and Kiikkala (1996), in their study exploring intra-operative surgical care in patients, found that the participants reported an appreciation of involvement in the decision-making process. They were less afraid of the surgery and were better able to participate in their care. Morse et al. (1994) link empowerment with enhanced comfort in patients, and Shultz et al. (1998), having researched antepartum and postpartum patients, record that patients found those nurses as caring who had helped them plan their care and discharge.

The first part of this chapter explores the way that experienced nurses describe the value they seem to place upon the encouragement of autonomy in their patients; it also describes some of the ways they empower them. The second part illustrates how student nurses see these notions of empowerment. The final section considers implications of empowerment and autonomy and suggests the limitations that may be present in embracing it as an overarching value in nursing practice.

Aspects of encouraging autonomy

It may be argued that issues surrounding the freedom and autonomy of individuals in society are becoming more and more prominent. This is reflected in healthcare too, and the encouragement of patient autonomy was a theme that emerged from the nurse transcriptions in this study. In Jack's caring scenario, he recounts a personal experience as a patient where he felt his personal autonomy was actually taken away by the nurse.

Jack: I think patients recognize if you are doing something to them or being with them. A good example: I went to A&E [accident and emergency unit] once, and I'd got my running shorts on and this nurse brought a card, she came and said, 'Do you want a blanket over you?' and I think that she must've thought that it was a caring thing to do. There were all these tables and I was on one, and I said that I didn't want a blanket, because I'd been running and I was warm, and she said, 'Oh, you really ought to have a blanket over yourself.' But I said that I was fine. She got embarrassed and put the curtains round, and I thought why did she do that? She completely ignored what I wanted, and what you are really doing is trying to demonstrate (a) that you can either care for me by providing some sort of cover or (b) maintain my dignity by pulling curtains round, but what you did was render me unautonomous ... I was chatting to George [a nurse experienced in A&E nursing] about it afterwards, and he said there are two types of nurses in A&E, and that's the one that carries the card and never does anything – they've got the card that demonstrates that they have got a patient. It was almost like I felt really ineffective in that situation as a person because I was fine; I had just got running shorts and a vest on. What's the problem with being laid on a table like that? I'd got my pants on and was decent, but you realize that she's not caring: she's trying to do things that *look* like she's caring.

Jack's example of being rendered 'unautonomous' clearly bothered him. He saw the nurse as someone who wanted to take something from him. This is an important observation, in so much as it may be argued that the nurse in order to care must do good for the patient. Patient choice – indeed, person choice – seems to be an increasing issue in modern society. It certainly seems to have a strong foothold in the movement of 'individualized care' paradigms established since the 1970s in nursing and healthcare in general. The provision of autonomy for patients seems to indicate a giving-back of power to the patient, which may imply that some elements of power and self-determination have been taken away.

Woodward (1998) carried out a study into professional caring. She finds that, in her sample, autonomy was seen as being a desirable aspect of how nurses cared for patients, and points out that autonomy has great emphasis placed upon it by the nurses in her study.

Anne's view of caring had quite a broad basis, but, again, patient empowerment was considered as being highly important; she also clearly identifies that it is not just nurses who can care.

Chris: What does the word 'care' mean to you?

Anne: I think it is difficult because what does caring mean and what is caring? It is a word that tends to get overused probably quite a lot, and nurses feel we have a monopoly on which I think is crap. I think that other people do care, other than nurses. I would say that it's looking after someone maybe in a situation that they feel unable to look after themselves but also appreciating that they may be able to do some aspects of what you are doing themselves and allowing them to do that or giving them the knowledge to do that. So I'd say it's definitely about providing the patient with something, but it's also about empowering that patient where possible.

Anne seemed to want to ease the patients' fear and anxiety by rendering them more autonomous and giving them more control about their care (again, it was seen as important to the nurse that her patient could be made more autonomous); her caring technique also seemed to be about teaching patients. It can perhaps be argued that providing information and teaching the patient are ways of actually empowering the patient.

Jill, who was a teacher prior to becoming a nurse, had this to say:

Chris: Do you think teaching and nursing have similarities?

Jill: Oh lots. To give the patients real independence and control of their own care, which is what modern nursing is about rather than doing everything for them, then you have to do a certain amount of teaching of patients in terms of health promotion, health education and in some cases teaching how to actually give physical care.

It seems that Jill considers teaching as a way to empower her patient:

Jill: Even within recovery, you can give a certain amount of responsibility back to the patients for themselves. When you are looking at analgesia, maybe when you first ask if they are in pain [and] they are not, you can say, 'I need to know when you are – tell me'; so they are then taking back the responsibility for themselves. So maybe it's that making them accept the fact that they are responsible for themselves and you are only there as a helper and assistant to give them their independence back.

Here Jill clearly points out that to her it is creating a real partnership with equality of power that shows care for the patient.

Jackie was a part-time practice nurse working in a single-handed GP's surgery. Jackie again saw the way she cared for her patients as a way to help them achieve greater independence for the future. Her work in general practice perhaps makes it easier to see that a community nurse's role is to give the patient as much independence as possible. Jackie discussed the satisfying parts of her job.

Chris: What is the most satisfying part?

Jackie: I think the most satisfying part is being able to get a person to adjust their lifestyle in a very small way that actually helps them be healthier and more effective really in their life in the long term.

I asked Cathy, the psychiatric nurse, what she thought were the main parts of her job. Amongst other aspects of care, she saw the encouragement of patient autonomy as being important in her care.

Chris: So what do you consider to be the most important parts of your job?

Cathy: Well, it would have to be lots of things because, as a psychiatric nurse, the most important things would be the relationships, communication, empathy and things like that. I'm quite interested in all the issues around being able to empower people because, obviously, if you work in psychiatry, you are dealing with a fairly downtrodden group of people in our society, so it's also really important to be able to make people have control and not feel controlled, and have choice and not feel as though choices are being made for them and be able to influence what happens to them and what happens in the service that they are part of, and things like that. I don't think it's new; it's just that there's a political emphasis on it now.

Chris: How much of that can you actually do in practice, or do things conspire against that kind of approach in psychiatry?

Cathy: I think that you can do an awful lot. I think that people tend to think of you as an empowerer in a big umbrella sense, in that you have got to have policies where somebody who is a service user is impacted on that, you've got to ... there's all these sort of things that are at government level, but just sitting listening to somebody is actually empowering them, and actually it gets right down to practical levels, where very often somebody is very agitated or distressed with mental health problems; they'll express emotions and maybe not in so many words they are not having any choices, and it may be as simple as somebody saying, 'Well, there are choices; let's look at what they are.' That's empowering somebody; that's allowing them to take their life forward rather than taking it forward for them, and it would all be based on good techniques. It's getting people to identify things in their lives, things that are important rather than making judgements about what you think it should be.

Cathy links empathy with empowerment; she also seems to have a strongly developed sense of justice and sees her patients sometimes as being very much at the powerless end of the spectrum.

The notion of power also plays a role in the ways that nurses perceive care and their role in the caring process. Some nurses see partnership as being important to a caring relationship; this can be a difficult thing to achieve between patients and nurses. There is a power gradient present between the two parties.

Some patients may not want to be equal partners; they may want to have some of the responsibility taken from them by the nurse. However, in the community, the relationship may be different from that in hospital. Perhaps the key to understanding a power relationship between patients and nurses is best understood by considering the nurses' view of relationships between them and the patient.

Pat is a practice nurse, but she reflects back to an earlier stage in her caring career as a midwife, and compares it to practice nursing.

Chris: So, it's a partnership?

Pat: I think the role that I am in now is probably more powerful than even when I was a midwife, which sounds crazy really because you think that somebody who's giving birth is solely dependent on their carer, but I think the reason that you are in a more powerful situation is for the same reason that the GP is in a very powerful situation. If you see a person week in week out, month in month out, year in year out, there's very little regarding their medical history and their social life and their family well-being that you don't know about. So, if I were to see someone for the first time such as yourself and saying 'I'm actually not very well but everything at home is fine', then you might say to me, 'OK, it may be that you have got a cold' or whatever. Whereas if somebody comes into my surgery and says, 'I'm having palpitations', they know that underlying behind all that is the evidence, so to speak, that you may think it's because their husband's left them, or you may think it's because they can't cope with their children, and I think that is a very fine balance, and you have to almost block out a lot of your knowledge: you almost have to unlearn a lot of what you know before you do your consultation.

Here Pat sees herself as being powerful, and the source of the power of which she speaks is related in her mind to the knowledge she has about her patient or about the situation that patient is in. It is about the power of care and caring. Pat is using her power to empower patients, not to dominate, coerce or control them. It is easy and perhaps trite to compare nursing's mainly female 'care power' with medicine's mainly male 'treatment power', and certainly beyond the scope of this thesis. As Benner (1984) points out, to define power or nursing exclusively in traditional masculine or female terms is a mistake. She states: 'To adopt a definition of power that excludes the power of caring does not gain the power of self-determination. Adopting coercive, dominating notions of power or strictly public relations abandons the value and commitments required for powerful caring and excellence.'

I asked Mike, the lecturer in oncology nursing, about care. He saw the encouragement of autonomy and empowerment not just for the patient, but also for their family, as being important:

Mike: Be able to talk to the relatives and involve them in the care as well. A nurse that doesn't impose themselves on the patients either, that can let the patient be himself or herself as much as you can within that sort of an institution. Be able to do things for the patient but also enable the patient to do things for themselves. In cancer care, it's very much the thing that's about enabling the patient to return as much as possible to their former life, and only they can do that, and so it's about you providing the resources for that person to do that.

Steve is a staff nurse in the intensive therapy unit (ITU); clearly patients there are usually extremely ill and generally unable to participate in their care. Steve spoke of encouraging independence in one of his patients despite the obvious difficulties of her critical illness:

> **Steve**: Lots of what I did for her when she was dependent was just making her comfortable and putting things close to where she could reach them, and serving her – yes, and being her servant in many ways – but she didn't look upon me as her servant or her dogsbody; she knew that I was doing that kind of thing so that she could reach them and in little ways being independent. I didn't have to feed her; I tried to encourage her to move her joints so that she could feed herself and that kind of stuff. Although it took a lot of time and effort, and, although it looked as though I was babying her in many ways and overly caring for her, it did move her forward, and it was the investment when she was particularly dependent that allowed her to move towards independence.

Encouraging independence seems to be something that can be quite a major thing, such as helping patients to make representation for what they see as unfair treatment, as in mental health care. Or it may be as simple as encouraging a patient to begin to feed him- or herself.

Ingrid, the ENT (ear, nose and throat) nurse from Denmark, also seemed to believe that an important part of her role was to promote a level of independence in her patients, although she acknowledged this was not always easy.

> **Ingrid**: If you take the tracheotomy again, patients and their families need to learn about how to actually clean off round it and make sure that it's OK. That's information as well. It's just there you have something to show them and you can teach them by letting them do it later on, but it's still information; it's no use just going in and doing it for them and saying this is how it is, and not telling them what it is they have to do and why.

To Ingrid, teaching was clearly a way to promote autonomy and not just to the patient but also to the family members as well. It was seen as important to build strong relationships to underpin attempts to empower patients. Ingrid went on to discuss what she saw as her primary role on the ward:

> **Chris**: What is the most important part of your job when you are on the ward?
>
> **Ingrid**: I tend to think it's providing information that is my most important job. But that's because I've been working with this particular kind of patient that normally could take care of their own physical needs and so therefore information became quite important to me because it is important that people who are being admitted to hospital know what is going on so they feel at least a little bit secure, and you follow up and keep appointments ... so that you [don't] say, 'Well, I'll come back in two minutes', and then you come back in half an hour.

Many patients want and actively seek out as much information as they can, relative to their condition or operative procedure, and that in itself is empowering. However, it is important that the nurse is sensitive to what patients really need. Some nurses may feel that they must give all information to the patient. Some patients may not want to know all the details of their illness or operation.

Later on, Ingrid described a situation from her past in the A&E department when she tried to educate and empower a child patient.

Chris: What gives you the most satisfaction at work?

Ingrid: It's satisfactory to see the work I am doing is actually working. I remember when I was working in accident and emergency there was this little boy, I think he must have been about seven, and a dog had bitten him, and he came in and he needed a tetanus vaccine. I tried to warn him ... I knew that it was going to hurt, and I told him that it would hurt a little bit but that I would try and do it quickly and gave him the right information at his level. This little boy had tears in his eyes, but he didn't cry and was quite happy that he didn't afterwards and that just made me feel that it was worth giving that information to that boy, and it was worth doing it this way.

Like their more experienced colleagues, students saw empowerment as an important way to underpin the care they gave.

Learning to empower

The significance of empowerment is seen in the words of Alice, a first-year student nurse.

Chris: In what ways do you care for your patients?

Alice: I try ... and help them through that, to be a guide and kind of be part of the process, to make decisions. You may not have a totally positive outcome, but you may be able to help somebody live with the situation. Be there for them. If somebody is given a diagnosis and said that you're going to die in six months, then that's a terrible thing; you've got to help them learn to live with that.

Alice, even with patients who are dying, saw empowerment as being a very real way to care for her patients.

Anton, a third-year student nurse, seemed to indicate that there were at times problems with being a student nurse who might want to empower patients.

Chris: What things do you find particularly hard in your day-to-day nursing?

Anton: Sometimes the people you work with, if you don't see things in the same way as them. Just a little example, for instance: instead of supporting somebody to walk to give them some independence to do it themselves and have somebody take over their [the patient's] role and they just do it for them.

Chris: It's often quicker, though, to put the patient's shoes and socks on than to wait for them to do it themselves.

Anton: If you help them too much, it's like you take that person's independence away.

Here Anton indicates perhaps some of the difficulty of promoting autonomy and independence as a student nurse; he also alludes to the problem of not having enough time to allow the patient to do things for themselves. This is arguably an increasing problem for all of those involved with providing modern healthcare.

Conclusion

There are real indications that nurses see the clear provision of patient autonomy as being a very important part of caring. This is also a theme that exists in some of the nursing literature relating to care. However, there may be some need for caution when attempting to empower patients. Woodward (1998), while stating that autonomy may be the new nursing mantra, seems to warn, however, that the race for patient/client autonomy may have certain drawbacks. Nurses need to be sensitive as to what the patient really wants, and autonomy may not be what all patients actually want or need. This must be balanced with the potentially uncomfortable problem of when patients remain powerless it may be that, even within the context of a 'caring' relationship, they will be persuaded to participate in clinical trials or consent to treatments which may not be in their best interests (Kelly 1998).

Campbell (1994) urges nurses to sensitively encourage emancipation, warning that the overemphasis of autonomy may in fact dehumanize health care and suppress moral agency. Woodward (1998) also urges that some discretion may be needed to protect patients from unfettered autonomy. She points out that ethical theory may identify the general principles that form the ethical basis of professional practice, but only through human relationship can the individual particulars become known. It is important that nurses are aware of the issues surrounding patient autonomy, because, as Riemen (1986) points out, in the past patients on admission have, on arrival to hospital, tended to forfeit control of what happens to them.

CHAPTER SEVEN

Giving of oneself

Introduction

Caring, it can be argued, is the essence of giving of oneself.

Nurses give to patients – of this there can be no doubt – time, energy and effort, and they spend time learning the skills and gaining the knowledge both as students new to nursing and also as students learning throughout their nursing career. It would seem, however, that there may be at least two quite distinct levels of care that can be given to the patient. The nurses in this chapter do not just describe the provision of physical care, though the interviewees do value this aspect: they seem to deepen the caring level by describing the giving-over of themselves. Here, perhaps, we can begin to appreciate the depth of emotional benevolence or commitment that nurses seem to provide for their patients. They arguably feel that to simply or mechanically provide care may not be enough; indeed, in their eyes to provide care without what might be termed 'genuineness' or something of themselves is to not adequately care for their patients.

It is on this question that Phillips (1996) wonders if nurses should be paid to smile. Could it be that by insisting that nurses always have a smile on their lips when 'doing for the patient', much like an air stewardess might have when attending to their passengers, patients might feel better cared for? She concludes, however, that, if this were to be the case, it seems possible that this would diminish their sincerity to the patients.

The link between motive and action is arguably linked, at least in the mind of the caring nurse. Perhaps the best nurses give the patient something of themselves.

The first part of this chapter considers the expressed views that describe the giving of oneself. It explores the physical and emotional aspects of care, and looks at the values placed on skills and knowledge by the nurse. The second part outlines the way that student nurses perceive some of the ways that experienced nurses give of themselves, and finally considers issues around skills and knowledge, and the relationship, in their eyes, between physical and emotional caregiving.

Aspects of giving of oneself

Linked perhaps with a view that nursing is something of a vocation, and that to care it may be that one needs to hand over or give something of oneself, Jack gives his personal definition of care. He certainly seems to see it as giving something of himself or giving something up.

> **Chris**: So what is care?
>
> **Jack**: I think care is about giving something up. Care is about giving up part of your self, whatever that might be. It could be time, energy, commitment to other people ... so I wouldn't say it's a physical thing or a psychosocial thing that's between two people. I think it's about you giving something up which a person either chooses to appreciate or not. So it's giving anything of yourself so that a person can benefit from it.

Later, on the question of paid caring, Jack speaks of committing something to the patient.

> **Chris**: What about paid caring?
>
> **Jack**: It is paid caring, but you can choose within that: it is paid from a very physical point of view – you give us this element of work and we will give you some money. However, a person can still choose whether or not they have given or committed some part of themselves to that or not, because they can go in and get the money, and we can provide physical care, but that doesn't necessarily mean to say that you have cared. There is the physical, paid element as well, but between two people there is something occurring – there is an element of giving something up.

While a distinction is made by Jack between paid and non-paid caring, there is still a view that the nurse, paid or unpaid, gives something to the patient. Later, he introduces the view that even if one is paid to care it does not seem to matter as long as the attitude is right. Then, at the end of this particular statement, he adds that anyone can give care or 'do for' a patient, but it is perhaps impossible to have proof that care was given in its true sense.

Jack describes a situation where what he did as a caring nurse – or, in his example, educationalist – really made a difference.

> **Jack**: From an educational perspective, I had a student once that got put in with a group that she really didn't want to be with, and it's almost like getting her to sit down and reflect on that: 'But what else is there?' So there's that element of sitting down with her and giving and stuff. So it's still about

giving something. In practice – what I always used to do. In that there's a push; this is not about the physical aspect of caring, but again it's still about giving something up.

When asked to describe her caring role in the PACU, Jill said this:

Jill: I give a lot of emotional support. You get patients who were anxious before they went in – because we often see patients before they went into theatre as well – and they are still anxious when they return from theatre, and you have to deal with that anxiety whatever it may be about. In some cases, it is feeling dreadful about being sick; they hate it. Feeling bad because they feel they are a burden on you. It can be hard, especially when you are busy – you have to personally dig deep!

Cathy, when interviewed, worked in psychiatric nursing, but she had previously worked as a general nurse. She, too, described giving something of herself in the way she cared for her patients.

Cathy: It's also this thing to do with dealing with a different sort of distress. It's just I find it really rewarding to work with people where you are having to give of yourself an awful lot.

She went on to compare general nursing with psychiatric nursing.

Cathy: The things that you do can't be based on 'Well, this person has had a stroke so they can't hold a spoon', so I do that bit for them, feed them. It's much more based on 'What can I give to that person in this state of distress?'; this person can't even talk they are so distressed, so what can I give of myself to make that meaningful for that person? I can help them psychologically through the situation. I can't help them to walk through it. I can't help them to feed properly. I can't do any of those things, but there must be other things I can do to make things easier, and they are all personal things, human things, to do with communication, touch and 'being there' sort of things, and I just find all of that much more rewarding for me.

These sentiments show that there is a clear feeling, at least with the nurses participating in this study, that they, in order to show and provide care, are giving something of themselves to the patient (or at least to the intervention). This giving of oneself seems to be present in both physical and psychological manifestations.

Physical and emotional aspects of care

Nursing has quite clearly a strong element of physical care attached to it; nurses often refer to it as 'hands-on' care. There is also, of course, an emotional element that is considered by some nurses as being equally, if not more important, to the giving of physical care to the patient. Lynn described the ways she valued mixing the physical and emotional aspects of care in her role.

Chris: What gives you the most satisfaction in your job?

Lynn: I like communicating with patients, and I like the hands-on, face-to-face talking, reassuring, caring, even the physical contact, helping someone put their shoes on, something as simple as that; people are so grateful for that. I think to do that you've got to understand how vulnerable they are as well.

Was it the physical or psychological aspects of care that Sue, who worked in theatres and recovery, valued most highly?

Chris: And you enjoy the hands-on care?

Sue: I do enjoy the hands-on care, but I also enjoy the other side of it. I feel it's very important to have somebody to listen to their worries, basically.

May, an experienced sister on an ENT ward, described what she considered to be 'good' nursing.

May: Basically, she's got to care, and I don't need highly technical, management-type nurses on this ward. I want somebody who can be able to care physically and emotionally for a patient.

Chris: What does 'care' or 'to care' mean to you?

May: To be concerned about someone else I suppose is the nearest thing to it and to give that concern action is to care physically and mentally.

Chris: What motivates you when you go out to give care, whether it is care for a student nurse or a patient?

May: I want them to be comfortable; that might be strange, but, if I come on in a morning and see somebody who can't really move properly and their neck's at an angle, I cannot resist; I've got to help them into that right position. If I come on and a student doesn't look too happy, I'm halfway between 'Do I respect her privacy?' and 'Do I ask her "Is everything all right – is there something you want to discuss?"'

Pat, a practice nurse, stated that in her role her patients in particular required a large level of emotional care from her.

Chris: What does caring mean to you, between you and your patients?

Pat: I would say care for me, and the clientele that I have at the moment, is approximately 80% emotional support, definitely. I do very little physical care, though it is, of course, very important.

From the above accounts, it is clear that the nurses clearly felt that two distinct but related aspects exist in the provision of nursing care, both equally important, but apparently important at different times to the nurse and patient.

What did Mike, the oncology lecturer, think care was?

Mike: If you show warmth and genuineness to them, I think that's important to them, that's what matters to them ... It's about enabling, being facilitative, being supportive – there's a whole list of adjectives like that. Also, you need to care for them in a very physical way, and if you do that in a close, caring way it can be more effective. I don't think you have to have all those things to be caring, but some of that mixture.

So Mike saw caring as a mixture of the two aspects: first, creating a bond or partnership and, second, providing actual physical assistance and nursing care to the patient. Mike's description here of the physical and emotional aspects of care seems to have an affinity with the issues surrounding giving of oneself, as described by Cathy in the earlier section. The next section considers the physical aspects of care as described by the nurses.

'Hands on'

There is a clearly defined and strong tradition of physicality and the provision of actual material care, in particular within the general nursing part of the profession. Intensive-care nursing is an area where nurses give a great deal of physical (intensive) care to their patients. Steve is a staff nurse in intensive care.

Chris: Is it the physical contact with patients that's important?

Steve: Yes, that is so important to be able to use your skills of practical nursing. I really value what I can do for the patient, but if it were just that kind of thing I wouldn't enjoy it. I think, again, it's the variety that makes it enjoyable: not being totally dedicated to looking after machines and being with all the technology and still being able to have hands-on stuff ... and interaction with the patients makes it all right. I could compare it with, say, working in the theatre, where the patients were totally unconscious and I didn't have too much to do with the patients, and it's more the machines than the patients, then that would be less enjoyable, I think.

Later on, Steve spoke about his own personal investment that he felt he had with patients.

Chris: You say it affects you more if you have a greater investment in the person?

Steve: There are a number of courses that it can progress along when it is developing. Sometimes we have patients that are unconscious on admission so there is no actual relationship ... So the only time the relationship develops then is when either the family makes their existence more meaningful for me by explaining, you know, 'She's a nice old lady, she likes her garden, she likes a cup of tea', those kinds of things, it then becomes a person, and in a way that's a relationship; or, if the patient wakes up and obviously they're conscious and they interact with me, then the relationship begins to develop. The relationship develops by me investing more and more in that patient, by being at the bedside with them [and] looking after them in a physical kind of way.

Here Steve points out the vital importance of practical and physical care in the provision of nursing; however, it seems that he believes that without an *emotional* aspect, care is incomplete. This supports the notion that care has two components which are of equal importance to the caring interaction; he too seems to be indicating that he is giving or investing something of himself in the relationship.

Giving of oneself and the physical and emotional aspects of care

Steve describes some of the complex issues surrounding the investment of emotion and physical effort in the patient. The two subcategories, 'Giving of oneself' and 'physical and emotional aspects of care', are described by Steve in the same section of interview.

> **Chris**: Could you give me your personal definition of care?
>
> **Steve**: I think it means to be concerned about something, for something to be important enough to you that you invest some effort in it emotionally and physically: to give of yourself. You initially need to be concerned about something for you to give that effort; so to me the actual care bit is a personal, intrinsic kind of thing. I think the actions that come from caring or being concerned about something you might be then asked to give of yourself, to invest some of your time, some emotional effort, that kind of thing. To me, it actually means for something to be involved, to care about it in that way.

Carla too seemed to identify that it was the mixing of the two parts of care which was important to the way she saw care.

> **Chris**: Could you give a personal definition of what 'care' means to you?
>
> **Carla**: I suppose it would mean looking out for every aspect of the person, so you are looking out for their physical needs, their personal needs, what they need to be that person that they are and looking beyond the extremities of the hospital environment or a healthcare environment.

It is apparent that to Steve and Carla investment of oneself is important, as providing both physical and emotional support to the patient is vital to ensure an adequate level of care. However, in the present healthcare system, skilful and knowledgeable practitioners of nursing are needed. This will be explored in the next section.

Using skills and knowledge

Nursing today can be an extremely technically demanding process: the nurse needs both to be able to function at a high level in terms of skilled competence, but also to be able to deal rapidly and effectively with a variety of difficult or even life-threatening situations; this ability is clearly important to some of the nurses in this study.

Chris: What part of your job gives you the most satisfaction?

Carla: In the acute patient episodes, for example; I have taken extra training to become someone who can give IV opiate, for example, and, if someone is in a very acute pain stage, the fact that you can actually get them through not only with the skills of giving somebody IV drugs but the fact that you can get them to deep-breathe, that you can stay with them, that you can actually commit yourself to some time and communication with them to use your skills, and get them out of that acute pain stage. When they actually say, 'Thank you, I feel a lot better now', then you think the world's a happier place.

Nurses are very powerful in the sense that they can provide vital physical care, such as in the example above, in the timely and effective application of analgesia. High-level technical knowledge arguably is seen as being powerful in nursing. However, it can be very simple things that can make a difference.

Mary also works in the PACU at a senior level.

Chris: What's important to you?

Mary: Little things: like post-anaesthetic-care patients have dry mouths and their lips are sore, and it's easy to get away from that; and little things like that really matter, I think.

Chris: What is the most important thing to you?

Mary: Safety initially, because it is a critical time. Safety first and then comfort, that leads to pain control, and I use pain-assessment tools to help that.

Chris: So getting them safe, getting them stable and then getting them comfortable? Because you have only got a fairly short period of time, haven't you?

Mary: Well, we keep them longer than some units. We keep patients that have had major ops for an hour, we get the beds up, we get warm blankets and we get them nice and comfy. We know what to do, and do it!

Steve, senior staff nurse in the ITU, found great satisfaction in using his nursing skills and knowledge to benefit his patients.

Chris: So what gives you the most satisfaction in your job?

Steve: I suppose one thing is orchestrating the whole team, and being able to manage the whole thing and utilize a number of skills, a lot of knowledge, and actually apply that to the patient, I suppose. As well as communicating, it's managing all the other things as well and having the feeling that you have managed a situation with lots of different demands and the need to utilize information and skills; that feels good.

Jane, the theatre sister, tried to imagine what it would be like for her to be nursed; she saw it in a personal way.

Chris: Can you give a definition of what 'caring' is to you?

Jane: Well, in my view if I'm caring for a patient as I would like to be cared for myself, to look after the basic needs, their safety, the mental perspective on what's going to be happening to them, and making sure that they are quite happy – happy is probably not the right word – but they are all right about what's going to be happening to them and making them feel OK about it.

Again, some of the nurses felt that, while using skills and knowledge was an important way to provide high-quality care for the patient, it was also seen as being vital that the skills and knowledge that nurses possess needed to be applied with a personal touch.

Combining skills and knowledge and the physical and emotional aspects of care

Jane works in theatres. This is a highly technical area, but she also values a caring and personal approach to her work, and she describes two aspects of care – the skills and knowledge, and the physical and emotional.

Chris: Technical skill, I suppose, is important because theatres are highly technical areas in which to work.

Jane: I think that they are basic skills that you need to have to be able to look after a person. I mean technical skills come with experience, but I think your basic caring, your personal approach, to people and things like that are a bit more important.

Jane looked back at her student days and recounted some caring memories; she was very proud of the skill that she and her team used, to care for one particular patient.

Jane: I remember when I was a student nurse I was allocated to a medical ward, and we had a lady who was unconscious. She came in at the beginning of my allocation and she was unconscious all throughout. We knew what to do, and we fed her and we cared for her, and she didn't have one pressure area at all, that lady, so that was an achievement, although there was no communication as such with her, but the actual caring part of it: there wasn't a mark on that lady when she came round, and I felt that we had looked after her.

This account of a caring memory from her student days seems to underline the importance that many nurses place on the practical skills that they possess, to care in a highly effective way, and this seems to be present in the students included in the study.

Learning to give of oneself

The students also seemed to be picking up on the importance of ways of caring from the experienced nurses that they had worked with on the wards. They too expressed the importance of caring for the patient in both physical and emotional ways.

Carl, the first-year student nurse, had begun to see certain ways of caring as important to the overall process. He had developed quite a sophisticated and reflective view of what care was to him. He identified two discrete factors of care: the physical and the psychological/emotional components that link in with the more experienced qualified nurses.

> **Carl**: I think caring is basically identifying what people's needs really are, and that's not only the physical need: it's all sorts of different other needs; I suppose psychological and emotional needs as well. The way I would see it is: care is very much an umbrella kind of idea, which has to deal with the specific and the general needs of the individual.

Carl seemed to be strongly influenced by more experienced nurses.

> **Carl**: But it's his or her ability [the nurses] as people to relate or get close to someone with a medical or psychological need. I'm always looking for good practice, and I mean everybody interprets their nursing role in a slightly different way. But I think there is a common thread, and I think ... they actually meet the need, in the most appropriate way for them.
>
> **Chris**: So what are the characteristics of a good nurse?
>
> **Carl**: It's what you as a person are like; in relation to others, I think, which is important. But it's being able to combine all the different skills, physical and emotional, which ... produce that sort of almost indefinable product really, and at the end of the day it's whether you can make a significant and substantial difference to the quality of that person's life that you're dealing with.

The students also seemed to see the physical aspects of care as being important and, again, were influenced by the qualified nurses' approaches to this aspect of care.

'Hands on': the students' perspective

Carl saw the actual physical aspects of care and caring as important. He also seemed to respect the qualified nurses who got involved in a practical way in caring for the patients on the ward.

> **Carl**: Well, the good nurse to me as well is the one that is prepared to muck in and to get their hands dirty and, you know, get hands-on experience and not be afraid to go and confront a situation, and not take refuge behind the nurses' station. I mean, I think we often use barriers in different ways to protect our sort of image ... unfortunately, I have to say this, but the more senior you appear to be in the clinical setting, the more temptation there is to stay your distance.

The observation of more senior or experienced nurses is a potent method of learning this role-modelling, which is clearly a factor here. Qualified nurses need to be aware of the ways that they act as role models to student nurses. Yam and Rossiter (2000) conclude that role-modelling is particularly important to the caring ethos in the clinical area (this would certainly be the case for Carl). The demonstration of a caring and positive attitude towards the patient enhances care. It may well influence the students' attitude towards a positive care approach in their future practice. They see strong and positive mentorship as highly influential to the care environment and to the way future carers developed.

Joan is a second-year student; again she seemed to point out that just to provide a blanket might not be enough: it seemed the motive was at least as important as the act.

> **Chris**: Do you think you can be effective in caring for patients without having that closeness to the patient?
>
> **Joan**: I think you do need a bit of both. I mean just doing something physical; I mean for someone who's cold and you just give them a blanket. You might consider that caring because you think that person can catch a chill, but that simple action, on its own, it doesn't actually mean anything at all; anybody can just do that.

Jess is a second-year student who seems to think there are two components of care, physical and emotional, with one more important than the other. I devised a scenario that might test her limits of care.

Chris: If you had knowledge that someone who you were caring for was, I don't know, had done horrible crimes to children or something like that, would that get in the way of you giving care?

Jess: No ... I don't believe it would prevent me from giving them physical care. It would be a mechanical care, I believe. That's ... how I may react. But I suppose it depends on the person's personality and how they are towards me, which would influence how I would act towards them.

Chris: So you'd be professional, you'd do the work?

Jess: I would hope I would do a professional job that I was meant to do and give the care that would be expected of me. But whether or not I would actually be able to care naturally? I believe there are two elements to care. There is the natural emotional care and then there's the physical, mechanical care ... which both come together to formulate care as a whole.

Chris: Which is the more important of the two?

Jess: The emotional care.

Jess indicates here that without an emotional commitment to the patient, the quality of the physical care provided might somehow be diminished or devalued.

Combining skills and knowledge, physical and emotional aspects of care and hands on: the students' perspective

Again, there were times that several aspects of care were described together, as in Jess's case.

Chris: Have you come across many things that have impressed you?

Jess: I have one that I saw whilst on a children's placement. There was a mum that was concerned about a young baby that had been admitted; he was showing signs of meningitis. The nurse that was dealing with her explained to her all the necessary procedures; she was clear, she was honest, she was concise and knowledgeable, but, as the sister was making her way out of the door, the mum said something that caught her attention and she turned around and she [the mum] just looked at her and said, 'Everything's going to be all right, isn't it?' And, obviously, she [the nurse] couldn't say that it was, but then she actually physically hugged the mum and the responses that she gave were caring and they were natural. And that really impressed me. Yeah, she just put her arm around her shoulders; she actually 'loved her'.

Here, all of the aspects outlined above were incorporated into a caring set of actions. Jess was clearly impressed by this. As Clayton (1999) points out, caring is a very important aspect of nursing care and is an aspect that may be forgotten in the rush of things. Nursing is seen as being more than just changing a dressing or taking vital signs. It is also about taking a few minutes to listen, to see the patient as a person, to hold a hand or hug the patient, to provide some comfort.

Anton, the third-year student, was asked what he thought was the best thing about nursing.

> **Anton**: Of course, first of all, it's to support the patients, to get them better. To help them achieve their independence.
>
> **Chris**: How do you do that?
>
> **Anton**: It's working together to achieve something, to give something of yourself to them.

Anton shared a caring situation he had had with a patient.

> **Chris**: Can you think of a situation, when you've cared for a patient, that sums up the caring?
>
> **Anton**: Well, the last one I can think of is, I was caring for a patient ... who was quadriplegic; he had an accident a year before he was admitted to the ward ... He lives in a nursing home, and he was admitted because he had an infection in his groin. Being a quadriplegic, he's got pain in his arms and legs so it's hard to move him, and we could – we did manage it with analgesia before ... I always wanted to work with him, during my shift; for example, he's got a special dressing I wanted to do and I wanted to understand him more, because with his condition, to be honest, there are staff who avoid him because it's hard work. I felt that I could give him something special.

Anton seems to be identifying what may actually be a therapeutic element of self (the nurse's self) that only he could give to the patient. This could perhaps indicate a developing self-awareness that as a nurse, by giving something of him- or herself, the nurse adds a significant level of value to the therapeutic, caring intervention.

Conclusion

Motive and action do certainly seem to be linked, in the minds of the nurses who shared their thoughts in this text at least. The first part of this chapter demonstrates some of the complexity that is intertwined in the caring process between patients and nurses. The link between physical action in the actual delivery of care to the patient and the creation of a solid emotional bond with the patient is important. This type of relationship often provides a deeply meaningful experience for nurses (Bertero 1999). It also may help them to give more effective physical care to their patients for, arguably, without a strong relationship between nurse and patient even the best and most motivated nurses will not be able to care for the patient as well as they otherwise might.

The student section in this chapter provides some identification that even newcomers to nursing quite early in their career begin to see that what might be described as the 'giving of oneself to the patient's needs' is a key way to enhance the caring process.

CHAPTER EIGHT

Taking risks

Introduction

At first, the phrase 'taking risks' does not really seem to be appropriate in a healthcare context. Taking risks in nursing is not about putting patients at risk by acting in a cavalier fashion or randomly experimenting with medications or nursing care; instead, the term is associated with pushing the boundaries of accepted care. It involves moving from the clearly defined boundaries that exist in any profession and developing new or innovative ways of, in the case of healthcare, caring for patients.

The first part of this chapter identifies how nurses seem to see that in order to improve the care they can give they need to push back the boundaries of care and even to challenge colleagues over the care they might give. In doing so, it considers notions of personal courage and patient advocacy. The chapter then looks at the nurses' ideas of challenge and the excitement they felt at times when caring. Finally, it outlines the ways that students learned to take risks when dealing with what they took to be sub-optimal care.

Aspects of taking risks

Jack seemed to believe that nurses who truly cared sometimes took risks in providing care.

> **Jack:** There's a difference between actively doing it, compromising somebody's care, trying to go out and give everything versus giving what you can under the constraints you've got. I think that when you are actively compromising care then you are letting yourself become uncaring. If you're giving everybody all the caring with the facilities that you've got, then that's fine. Because if you are really delivering care, then you are not worried about what you do.

The above account indicates that an element of courage is required to care for one's patient in a perhaps more radical way. The courageous nurse is one that, in order to care fully, in the nurse's view, meets the patient's needs in what some nurses might consider to be a deeper way.

Fagerstrom et al. (1998) in their research exploring patients' and nurses' perceptions of caring, describe this kind of nurse as one who is fully aware of the patients' physical and spiritual suffering, and has the courage to 'meet' the patient. In Fagerstrom et al.'s view, everyday small talk with the patients is not enough; the nurse must have courage to face patients' difficulties, like anxiety, insecurity, uncertainty and depression.

Nurses do not work in isolation from other groups of nurses or health-care professionals. Practice nurses in their daily nursing often work closely with other members of the multi-disciplinary team; I wondered what Jackie's view was of her part of that team. Jackie described how her way of caring for the patients sometimes differed from some of her colleagues'.

> **Jackie**: I work differently to the other nurses. The other nurses tend to work perhaps like I did when I was a staff nurse in the hospital, very much by rules and regulations and not forwarding themselves; although they are doing the studying, they seem to be going in a very regimented sort of way. I feel I do work more in the ways of the private people I come across: some of the physios, some of the acupuncturists and counsellors who decide what they need in a job and work for the patients and not to how the institution says you ought to work.

Here Jackie seems to be identifying what might possibly be a different approach to care between hospital and the community setting. What about differences between general nursing and psychiatric nursing?

Cathy, the only psychiatric nurse in the interviewed group, also saw her role in caring as one that at times required her to make a stand for her patient and sometimes to take risks. I asked Cathy to describe a caring situation from her practice.

> **Cathy**: One example would be a manic-depressive lady who functioned like you or I 90% of the time and had a holiday in Spain once a year, and while in Spain was drinking alcohol as well as taking lithium, so got flown back on an emergency flight halfway through her holiday, and landed and ended up in quite a manic state. It was almost to the date every year she would come into hospital. I remember looking after her, and one psychiatrist who was fairly new to the service insisted that this lady not only had lithium but also had an injection of a psychotropic medication and had more or less steam-rollered this woman into having this injection, and it was on the prescription card to be given; and I remember being in the situation where I was in a human sense dealing with this lady who was really high and unable to concentrate, and all those other problems, and her communication was a bit disrupted but was really saying, 'I don't need that injection. I don't want it. I just need

not to drink, calm down and keep taking the lithium.' I ended up refusing to give the injection against the psychiatrist's wishes, and this went on for a number of weeks, and there were some really difficult issues around stopping the other nurses giving the injections, because the minute you leave your shift and it's on the prescription card, somebody else might just go and give it, and this lady wouldn't be in a position to say not to. I was trying not to set up a conspiracy against this doctor but at the same time be an advocate for the woman. We ended up not giving her the depo [slow-release medication]. She got better and went home on lithium, and I've seen that lady numerous times after her summer holiday since and she always remembers. I've had loads of situations like that where you put yourself out on a limb and think you are going to be in a lot of trouble, but in actual fact you know in your heart of hearts what you are doing is right.

Cathy took a risk in the professional sense in not obeying the doctor's order to give the injection. It is hard for a nurse to refuse a medical order; however, it is sometimes essential in order to protect the patients from harm.

Steve, the ITU staff nurse, felt that sometimes going that step further or stepping out of what was normally done for his patients was important to his caring.

Steve: A lady that I looked after sticks in my mind for many reasons. She reminded me a lot of my mum, and I'd looked after her for a period of months in intensive care, as opposed to the usual as she to'd and fro'd between the ward and intensive care a few times, and she was a nice person that I built up a relationship with, and the family were nice, and I built up a relationship with them as well. I managed to build up a relationship with her; she was critically ill and sedated for a long time, and, as she woke up and moved more towards health and independence and getting off the ventilator, for example, I built up a good relationship with her, and she trusted me a lot, which was important, and the family did. We did get her better, which was obviously the goal, and moved her to the ward, and I was allowed to do lots of the things for her that I think are important and helped get her back to health and wellness. For example, she was in when the unit was particularly quiet and when we moved her to the ward the unit remained very quiet, so on the day when there was nothing much doing and we got some spare time, myself and the physiotherapist, who had become quite close to her as well, used to take her for walks round the hospital grounds in a wheelchair, and to me that upped her spirits. From when she became conscious the whole thing that kept her ticking along and motivated her to get well and get home was the view that she was going to get better and was; on the times when everything seemed monotonous, it was just somehow changing things. And when she was quite depressed on the ward and we went up and spent some time with her and talked to her, took her out and gave her a change of scenery when she wouldn't have been able to do that, those were the little things that just changed the direction of her recovery in some way. That's certainly not typical of what we normally do for patients but in many ways characterizes our relationship, and what we did should be the characteristic of nursing, even if it's in a small way.

Steve showed that, in order to care fully for his patient, he left his unit to give extra care to his patient, despite the fact that she was now the responsibility of another group of nurses on another ward. This is very atypical of accepted nursing and clearly crosses the normally defined boundaries of care.

Mary, the sister in PACU, also believed that it was important sometimes to step beyond the normal parameters of care for patients.

> **Mary**: Also sometimes I think nurses don't know when its OK to maybe use their own initiative and not follow protocol. I think some nurses are very protocol-based, and they are either unconfident or unwilling or for whatever reason don't bend protocol; they don't bend a procedure. Your experience or initiative should tell you when you maybe don't have to follow procedures, because every patient is different.

Ingrid described a situation from her practice in which she took something of a risk with one of her patients.

> **Ingrid**: I remember one particular patient who was illiterate (with a tracheotomy), and that was a huge problem. This was someone who used to take care of his wife. She wasn't very bright and couldn't take care of herself in society, and she was quite a few years younger than he was, so he was used to being in charge. But he was illiterate [but] in his mind he still needed to take care of her at home, but he was in hospital. We speeded up the process of getting his speaking tube in much faster than normal; that was the only way. It was a risk but one we needed to take; you could see, when he got upset or if he was unhappy about what you did, he got very frustrated and anxious. We just had to speed up the process to where we could get him speaking and able to feel he was in control.

The extracts from the above accounts clearly indicate that some nurses feel it necessary to, at times, make a stand against their professional colleagues' interpretations of normal nursing procedures or protocols in the course of caring for a patient. As a consequence of these risks being taken, nurses face risks ranging from being looked upon as unusual by their colleagues to possibly being held professionally accountable for not following an order. If nurses perceive their peers' care as being less than optimal, in their eyes at least, it becomes an ethical and professional dilemma in practice. Arguably, nurses then need the courage to confront and deal with these issues to benefit their patients' needs, and in doing so must push the boundaries of commonly accepted caring and take risks.

Some nurses shared their feelings during their interview relating to the excitement they sometimes felt in their jobs. They enjoyed being stretched professionally; they seemed at times to take considerable pride in using their technical excellence and ability to work under pressure in providing what they saw as highly focused and quality care for their patients; this is described in this study as 'getting a buzz' from caring.

Getting a buzz

Working in a busy acute ward or department in a hospital can be an exciting experience. Anne works as a manager in theatres for half of her work time and as a teacher for the other half. One of the reasons she enjoyed theatre work was for the excitement that it brought her.

> **Anne**: I liked the cut and thrust of it. I liked the emergency side: you didn't know what patients were coming in, what would be expected of you. I like the patient interaction, but I like the technical side as well, along with working with the multi-disciplinary team, so it wasn't just nurses. There would be ODAs [operating department assistants] and the anaesthetists and the surgeons ... it was quite dynamic ... I just liked the prioritization of the care that was needed, and the demand. I felt it really benefited the patient, even though they were not usually aware of it!

Jill (a teacher in the past) spoke of 'getting a buzz' from her nursing.

> **Jill**: Yes, it gives me a buzz to be able to look after somebody and know at the end of it, which is another reason why I chose a theatre environment, because you know at the end of it 99% of your patients are going to feel better. It gives you that buzz to say, 'Yes, I have helped. I have been beneficial. I have been of some use to the patient.' When you have got somebody come from theatre who is in agony and you know you can deal with that agony and make them feel comfortable so that they can deal with all the other problems that having an operation entails, then, yes, you feel great.

Jane, the theatre sister, also seemed to enjoy the uncertainty and excitement in her role. She was telling me, as part of her caring narrative, about a patient who had a leaking abdominal aneurysm:

> **Jane**: In theatre I had a chap a few months ago [who] was frightened. We were talking and he went off [his condition rapidly worsened]; he wasn't quite out of it, and the adrenaline starts to go, and you know you've got to get him down and get it repaired, and the outcome was good; so that's another aspect of theatre work that I like. It's the not knowing what's going to happen. To do that and have him rushed in and organize people and get it all done and then he's in recovery. People have turned round and said that was good because you sorted everybody out, everybody knew what they were going to do and it all came together, and it makes me feel 'You're a giant'.

In common with excitement and being stretched, it seems that the challenge of providing quality care is also an important aspect of the caring process for some nurses.

Challenge

Steve, the senior staff nurse in intensive care, seemed to enjoy the challenge of overcoming difficult situations.

Chris: Why intensive care?

Steve: It's varied, it's rapidly changing, and I like that element – that it's not monotonous, although perhaps aspects of it are. It has become more enjoyable through being able to handle the challenge better. If I was the sort of person who wasn't calm and wasn't able to operate in those situations, I don't think it would be enjoyable at all, and I couldn't care for the patients properly. Part of the enjoyment and satisfaction comes out of being able to manage it and handle it and not just the fact that something's happening acutely and things are out of control.

Mike also expressed personal enjoyment from the challenge of working with, in his case, cancer patients.

Mike: It's never the same: no two patients are the same. OK, treatments can be similar, but the psychosocial responses are always completely different. Patients come from completely different backgrounds; that's the exciting part, dealing with different patients, having to change your approach to how you care for them. Some patients like to talk about it [their diagnosis]; other people go into denial, and, again, it's about how you actually deal with all those different reactions which is really challenging.

The above accounts describe what the respondents value and enjoy in their roles. It is arguably about professional pride in their work and says a lot about how they perceive the caring nurse's role to be in practice. The students, however, perhaps owing to the fact that they were not expected to deal with critical situations in their training courses, did not highlight 'getting a buzz' and 'challenge' as being a significant part of the ways that they understood care. They did, however, in their interviews state the need to, at times, be courageous and to sometimes take risks, a requirement which they saw as being an essential part of caring for patients. In their cases, 'taking risks' seemed to mean their standing up for those patients whose care was less than what (the students felt) they deserved.

Learning to take risks

Alice, although a student nurse in her first year, had at times stood up for patients when she felt that they were not being cared for in the right way.

> **Alice**: I think the key to good care is being strong enough to object if you don't agree with something.
>
> **Chris**: That's not always easy, is it?
>
> **Alice**: No. Not as a student, no.
>
> **Chris**: Have you ever had to make a stand?
>
> **Alice**: Yeah; it's not easy. It's not at all. I just had to voice my opinion of what was happening and consider what the consequences of me not speaking out would have been for that person. It took a lot of guts to speak up, because I'd not been there that long. And I felt that I didn't really know as much as these other people about the situation, but I just felt that I had to say something.

This account shows that having to make a stand against something that the student nurse feels strongly about is not always easy. As a student, it is very hard to go against the established members of the ward team. They not only have the ability to make life difficult for you but also can fail you practically by giving you a poor report. Carl also at times had felt unhappy with the care he had witnessed being given by the senior staff; as a student it can be extremely hard to speak up against qualified staff. In this extract, he recounts how he felt that qualified nurses could have given more.

> **Carl**: I have had occasions where I felt afterwards there was definitely an opportunity to go beyond sort of purely clinical aspects of care. And actually to spend some time, real quality time, maybe just talking, chatting, listening to the patients.

It is not always the fear of being given a poor report that prevents a student from speaking out against what they might see as sub-optimal care; sometimes students do not have the professional basis of knowledge or the confidence to do so, as in Carl's case here.

> **Carl**: You do feel rather impotent sometimes. You think, on reflection, I had the opportunity to sort of pitch in and say something there.
>
> **Chris**: How exactly do you feel in those situations?
>
> **Carl**: I feel quite frustrated when I see these things happen, but I say to myself, 'Well, of course, I'm not a qualified nurse', and I mean if I were in that same situation, under that kind of pressure, would I react in that way? You know, perhaps, if I'm realistic about it, perhaps this is what the nursing experience is actually like in the real world. But there have been occasions when I've felt like ... trying to be the patient's advocate, if you like, but holding back for various reasons.

Chris: Holding back?

Carl: Not wishing to intrude on professional prerogatives really. Yeah; so it's not easy.

Carl also was impressed with different ways of caring he had seen, stepping out from the normally accepted nursing approach; again it is an indication that role-modelling can be a very powerful means of learning to nurse and care.

> **Carl**: I had an experience not long ago working as an auxiliary on a surgical ward and ... it was very, very quiet, but the person I was allocated to was in fact a fairly newly qualified nurse and he was on the drugs round and I'd been on a 30-minute break. [I asked him if he had finished the round yet.] And he said, 'No, I've not actually. I've been sitting talking to patients and having a little chat with them and chewing the fat, and just basically having a good listen to them really.' And I thought, 'Well, good for you', you know? That's not what you normally see. That's to my mind very, very caring and a responsible attitude to carry into the ward, but that was just a small incident really in many ways, but I thought it was quite a refreshing sort of approach.

From Carl's interview, I think you can begin to see some of the difficulties that a student nurse might face when observing uncaring nurses while upon their placement. This can be traumatic and perhaps damaging in the long term to students.

Paula, the third-year student, described how she took personal responsibility to find out further information in order that she could help her patient more fully to recover.

> **Paula**: I got to know a patient on a medical ward, and, on first appearances, it seemed that nothing [the various treatments] was working at all. They were trying everything that they possibly could to help this woman. I tried to look deeper into the issue that was affecting her and what I found shed a whole new perspective on her care. I think that if more nurses did that then you wouldn't go round in circles as much and patients would be seen in a different way and approached from different perspectives.
>
> **Chris**: So you were actually doing that bit extra so you could care for her better? You looked at things slightly differently?
>
> **Paula**: I mean it's all right just saying to the patient, 'I've called the physiotherapist', but you need to take responsibility to actually sit down and talk to the patient and figure out what she thinks.

Paula here has taken a great step forward in identifying that to her the nurse must take responsibility to go the extra mile to care for patients in a fuller way than perhaps might be considered normal. This, from my point of view, is a very satisfying thing to hear from one so new to nursing; there are not many experienced nurses, from my observations, who show such motivation to look at other ways to help meet the patients' needs in the way Paula did.

Conclusion

Issues relating to taking risks indicate that some of the nurses in this study see that in order to provide a high standard of care they must at times step out of the normal parameters of nursing care. The culture of nursing tends to be rigid and even constricting in the ways it makes nurses conform to its protocols. What we are really talking about here is how nurses want to change or move their caring onwards, in order to encourage what Benner (1984) describes as 'transformative care'.

I believe that nurses do need to push out from positions of professional safety and begin to take risks for their patients. Transformative caring is epitomized by a nurse's desire to release the patient from their prescribed role.

CHAPTER NINE
Supporting care

Introduction

In this chapter, the nurses identify the fact that they believe there are certain essential factors required to ensure that care can be delivered effectively. The first section considers the importance of the creation and maintenance of support systems of work, both in a physical (managerial and systems of command and control) and a psychological (counselling and support) sense. The second part describes the importance of strong commitment and well-defined ideals as essential to the provision of good care. The final part explores how students view commitment, and highlights how they value support from colleagues when they encounter difficult situations in their caring for patients.

Caring for colleagues

Anne, for half her time, is a clinical coordinator in the operating theatres, with managerial responsibility for her team. Anne's priorities for care seem to incorporate a wider, more encompassing view. She feels that to provide good care to the patients, her staff members need caring for as well so that they might do their jobs better.

> **Anne:** The first thing from a priority point of view would be the care of the patient, but thereafter my role is definitely to make sure that the staff are OK; that's this old adage of 'Who cares for the carers?', and I don't think a lot of people do, and I don't think we are very good at caring for each other. I think we are very good at looking after patients and very sympathetic towards patients, but if we have colleagues that are ill we find that very stressful. I've joked sometimes and said that part of my role is definitely that of social worker: it's listening to people, how they feel, what their problems are.

Anne spoke of the difficulty of providing care sometimes; here she describes how nurses need to be supported in their caring role.

> **Anne**: Caring for someone is hard work, and it demands a lot of attention, and you perhaps need support yourself while doing it. I don't think that that is noted in some areas. I think it's felt that it [nursing] has always been a vocation and nurses are superior beings that can cope with anything, and that's not true. They do need support themselves, and I don't think the support network is there when they're providing this care all the time.

Yam and Rossiter (2000) support this view; they found that nurses considered the provision of a supportive environment as being essential to ensure care for the patient. They too found that cooperation and support for colleagues in the clinical setting helped achieve the best possible care for the patients in need.

Jill, again from theatre, thought that the creation and maintenance of teamwork was important in supporting the process of care. In her caring scenario, she recounted the impending death of a patient after an operation.

> **Jill**: You've still got patients to care for, but you've got this dying patient and their family to look after, so it's giving them the time, the privacy, the seclusion. Included are things like trying to get the patient round fairly quickly, onto a ventilator, onto our equipment in recovery and making the patient presentable, basically. Getting rid of things, the bloodstained sheets and theatre gowns, making sure that any unpleasantness about surgery wasn't on open view. The patient's family shouldn't have inflicted on them the sight of an actual surgical incision and the dressings and the fact that there was blood still leaking from the incision and things like that. It worked, but only as a team. There were some doing tidying up, the cleaning up and making comfortable of this patient who was dying. There were members of the team seeing the family, preparing them and bringing them in and other members of the team looking after the other patients who were coming out of theatre to go back to wards. So there was a lot of emotional input, and at the end of it, it needed time for us all to sit down and deal with the emotional input to each other as well.

Jill outlines here a traumatic and difficult situation in practice. Jill and the team wanted to make things as right as possible for the family members in a tragic situation. She states clearly that, in her view, time was needed to get the team members together and support each other. This can be seen as a way of ensuring that nurses are able to sustain a caring ethos in practice; for this, Jill believes that a supportive environment is needed.

Some nurses hold that a major part of their caring role is the creation of a caring environment. Lynn greatly enjoyed the caring one-to-one contact she had with her patients but also pointed out that it was vital to have a system of organization in place to support care.

Lynn: Dealing with patients, that's obviously the most important part, but what I'm learning more and more is that I love that side of it. I love that contact, and I love making patients feel welcome and that they are being looked after properly, but increasingly there's problems with actually getting systems of work in place so that can occur, and increasingly I'm looking at these important things. One of the important things is actually having a system of work on a ward that allows that [care] to happen, and increasing problems are little things that really distress patients and us that are caused through systems of work not being in place, that things can actually work to benefit patients. A lot of the time it's just patients distressed and suffering because systems of work aren't in place. If you haven't got the patient central to the organization work, then they are suffering.

Lynn clearly felt very frustrated at the way the system ran at times. She could not give the patients the care she clearly felt they deserved. This is reflected in the literature by Tuck et al. (1998), who describe the importance to a caring organization, such as a hospital, of the creation and maintenance of a strong and well-organized system of care management. In addition, they state that: 'The type of health and nursing care provided within an organisation reflects the philosophical view of the administration.'

Lynn went on to talk about change within the system.

Lynn: We've just done a multi-disciplinary audit to get more painkillers for people at home, and the fact that you can actually move systems of care to benefit patients gives you an even bigger sense of satisfaction ... that something that I've done has got patients better painkillers at home, and that involved an enormous amount – two years – of work; that gives me enormous satisfaction because it's the patients benefiting that matters, and they have, through a major project, and it's the change that matters to me. It's the improvements to the system that's important.

Clearly, if one is creating a caring system, a large part of the efficient running of any system is the maintenance of good communication. Carla, a staff nurse in the PACU, highlighted this aspect of care support:

Carla: Communication! Communication with the patients to get them out of pain and get them through a difficult period, communication with your colleagues to support you and support them and communication with management, otherwise everything falls down.

Mary was quite senior in the PACU; she too thought that creating an environment that supported the carers was important to the overall provision of high-quality care:

Mary: I enjoy the management side of it. I get ... 'bored' is an awful word to use – but it's all gynaecology patients, and it doesn't personally stretch me as much as it could. This is why I'm always interested in doing courses and doing all these projects and stretching myself in those respects. I enjoy the personnel side of it. I like managing a team of staff and helping them to make things as they should be. I prefer the management side of things, the humanistic side. I enjoy dealing with staff, and I enjoy researching different projects: anything that would help development and care within the unit to improve it.

Mary sees managing the system as important; this may be influenced by her seniority. As a senior nurse, her focus has perhaps moved from the individual patient to the strategic issues in caring, and her position has the authority to do this. Jane is a sister in theatres; she echoes Mary's view.

Jane: The health and safety of the patient, of course, and I think keeping the team together. Motivating the team, making sure they are happy at their work and that things get done properly.

The above accounts all show a well-defined appreciation of the need to ensure a well-organized system that will help ensure care is delivered in an efficient way. The nurses who described this aspect as important to them unsurprisingly tended to be the more senior nurses with a greater management role in their work.

Rayman et al. (1999) argue that nurses today are finding the environment of practice more stressful and less supportive. This is despite the signs that organizational norms are changing in ways that seek to accommodate more fully the concepts of care and autonomy. Paradoxically, they see one exception to this as being professional nursing cultures. As they point out, in order to begin to create a more supportive and caring culture in healthcare, organizational and professional norms of caring need to be built with congruence between the stated values and the demonstrated values.

Commitment

It is perhaps obvious that healthcare professionals need to show a high level of commitment to patients in their work. Without this, some felt that high-quality care was often compromised. Mary described her attempts to get her team to maintain their motivation.

Mary: Getting members of our team to still remain interested, that's something I've found hard. A lot of them have worked there a long time. They think that what they do is OK, and it's pretty hard to get people to change. There are some nurses I've seen who don't seem bothered, and I just think they are doing more harm than good.

Having commitment is arguably akin to having strong ideals; these two sub-categories were sometimes expressed together.

Commitment and ideals

Lynn, a staff nurse, saw commitment and the possession of ideals of caring for the patient, and to caring in general, as being very important.

> **Lynn**: I do think you have got to want to be able to help people; you must have some sort of commitment and ideals – you have to have some desire to help people who are vulnerable.

Steve is a senior staff nurse in ITU; he described his ideals and commitment to providing the best kind of care but also illustrated some of the frustration he feels when others around him do not match his levels of commitment.

> **Steve**: The things I get most annoyed about usually come from my interactions with other people, usually nurses and doctors. I usually rationalize it by saying, 'Well, I fall out with the people that I live with and I love; so I'm going to fall out with the people that I spend this amount of time with at work, and I don't necessarily get along with [some of them] too well.' If I think something can be done, and it isn't done and things aren't optimum. Perhaps I'm a bit of a stickler, but, if things are not optimum and I see that there has been a lack of care or effort, I don't like that. People who don't necessarily care, who are a bit cold, that kind of thing.

Carla too described her strong commitment to the patients and to her role as well.

> **Carla**: Because communication skills are so very, very personal – and you can't go knocking other people's – they have to, I hope, that they would learn [these communication skills] by example. With junior nurses, I'll mug them and get them to do this – student nurses, anyone. People will say, 'Oh, there goes Carla, and she's doing her relaxation therapy: she'll have them huffing and puffing in the aisles.' I don't care, they can jest ... because, as far as I'm concerned, I am committed to giving good service to those patients, and, if I'm on the other side, I want that service.

Carla does not seem to worry about her popularity; she just wants to do a good job in caring for her patients. Amongst other things, Jane saw commitment to caring as essential:

> **Chris**: What makes the best kind of nurse?
>
> **Jane**: Somebody with quite a bit of understanding, patience. Being committed to the patient, being able to communicate, just to tell them what is going on, to have that knowledge.

Ingrid (an ENT staff nurse), despite not really wanting to nurse at the beginning, had developed very high standards in her care.

> **Ingrid**: If I can have the circumstances around it that I want to. If I don't find the work I'm doing is good enough or living up to the standards that I want it to live up to, I'm not satisfied.
>
> **Chris**: So am I right in saying you have got very exacting standards?
>
> **Ingrid**: I don't know if I have. I just want to live up to them, the standards that I've got. If I don't do that, I just don't feel I'm caring for the patients properly.

It is hard not to be impressed by the ways that the nurses described their commitment to their patients. Nurses need to be highly motivated to do their jobs to the best of their abilities. Nursing is an occupation that is always highly demanding, and to maintain the initial idealism that the nurses above have indicated that they still have for nursing is very rewarding to find. The students also showed their motivation and commitment in similar ways to their more senior colleagues.

Learning to become committed

Students often seem to come into nursing with high levels of commitment to caring. They also can have highly developed ideals. Learning to care, however, is clearly an aspect of care that is an important part of the educative process for many students.

I asked Carl, a first-year student with strong Christian beliefs, to describe his commitment to nursing.

> **Carl**: I feel that, philosophically speaking, there is a very strong link between the vocational sort of approach and commitment and the whole process of nursing – and what nursing is attempting to do. I really feel that there is an implicit link between the values and the principles that are espoused by religion and the caring sort of ethos of nursing and its essence.

Students, it would seem here, are often upset by difficulties and emotional stress in their nursing education and early exposure to patients in their practical nursing experiences, especially perhaps when qualified nurses do not show a commitment to care. This will be examined further in the next chapter.

Generally, nursing can be upsetting and very difficult at times; this is perhaps worse for newcomers. Some of the students referred to times when they had felt overcome by events on the ward. One of them saw it as essential for nurses to provide support for one another in times of emotional stress.

Joan described a situation where she became extremely upset following a saddening interaction with a patient but was clearly glad to be supported by a more senior colleague.

> **Joan**: I kind of walked out of the room because another nurse came in, and I quickly said goodbye to the patient and walked out of the room, and I started crying outside the room. But I did actually feel quite ashamed after that because it was 'Oh God; I can't believe I was so weak,' you know? I could have waited until after my shift because I only had half an hour before my shift ended. But the staff nurse was really ... so good.
>
> **Chris**: Did she pick up on the fact you were sad?
>
> **Joan**: Yeah. Well, I started crying my eyes out. I think as soon as she put her arms around me, and I responded and cried even more actually. I don't know why but it just made me feel ... she could understand. To me, her body language was saying that I can understand how you feel, and that's why it made me cry even more.

Paula, the third-year student nurse, believed that support between nurses was important in caring for the patient.

> **Paula**: You can't leave them if someone's upset about something, then it's important for the ward and the patients – isn't it? – if you take into account the other nurses' needs as well. I think one of the downsides to care is if the team is not supporting you.

From a student's point of view it is impossible to think of a more potentially damaging factor than not providing an effective support mechanism to help them understand and come to terms with the difficulties and emotional assaults that they encounter in their formative years in nursing. What this does seem to show is the ways that student nurses learn from their more experienced mentors. If support is not provided in a timely and effective manner for them, there must be a danger that the students, in time, may not provide the caring support which is so necessary for care, thus worsening what may be described as being a cycle of emotional damage in nursing. This will be explored in the next chapter.

Conclusion

It is important to ensure that care is supported in whichever ways possible. The nurses in this study felt that a supportive environment was an important way of promoting care within the practice. Nursing is a complex and emotionally challenging occupation; it is essential that nurse administrators identify this fact and ensure that management philosophies reflect this requirement. It is not an easy task to make happen; financial constraints restrict managers in common with the nurses at the bedside. In fact, operational managers are even more aware of these restrictions. However, as Sanford (2000) points out, the ability to combine caring with understanding, and balancing the needs of customers, employees, organizations and managers is the hallmark of a loving leader. Supporting these sentiments, Nortvedt (2001), when considering the moral considerations in nursing care, points out that in a healthcare system in which distribution considerations are crucial, practising nurses must provide for both actual and potential patients' access to relational care.

In helping nurses to provide high-quality care, Bassett (1999) identifies the urgent need to provide a strong level of emotional support to practising nurses at the interface with patients. He sees the provision of a widespread network of clinical supervision, by nurses for nurses, as a key way of helping nurses overcome the physical and psychological demands that nursing brings with it.

McQueen (1997) states that the significance of the emotional nature of nurses' work is beginning to gain more recognition in the literature. Stress and burnout are increasingly common themes in nursing literature. Nurses, wherever they work, need support to help them maintain their ideals and commitment in practice. This requires mutual support between nursing teams and individuals and, in addition to this, organizational support systems need to be available to nurses.

CHAPTER TEN

Emotional labour

Introduction

The theme of 'emotional labour' is one that is unique to the students included in this study; it seems to reflect the emotional challenge of learning to nurse, and may be magnified by the sometimes painful transition that can occur when moving towards qualified-nurse status (Bassett 1994a). It is unlikely that this concept is unknown to the more experienced nurses in the study (perhaps, though, it may be forgotten), but it was the students who described it most clearly in their interviews. It is also undoubtedly the case that this phenomenon exists outside the traditional caring occupations (Henderson 2001).

'Emotional labour' is a term that describes the often very difficult things that nurses are expected to do in their daily work. Hochschild (1983) uses the term 'labour' instead of care in her research into flight attendants, because of the nature of their work (smiling, being friendly, kind, courteous etc.). She defines 'emotional labour' as the induction or suppression of feeling in order to sustain an outward appearance that produces in others a sense of being cared for in a convivial, safe place. Bolton (2000) describes it as a form of emotional management or control designed to enhance care. I have used it here as I feel it sums up very well the ways that students seem to, first, be affected by the raw emotion sometimes present in caring for a patient and, second, because the expression of the raw emotion is quite often for various reasons suppressed by the student.

It is often hardest in many ways for students to deal with these emotional assaults on themselves, as they will not have developed ways of dealing with these issues as their more experienced colleagues and mentors may have. Smith et al. (1998) support this view and describe several situations where nurses 'had issues' that were of importance to students. One nurse stressed the importance of knowing where to draw the line in nurse–patient relationships. Another described nurses as actresses who left their 'personal self' at the ward door before going on 'stage' in the ward. A third nurse described how she suppressed any negative feelings she had about patients when relating to them. These examples from the literature show that nurses can bury their own feelings to either protect the patient or protect themselves from perceived harm.

The student nurses in this book describe similar painful or difficult situations from their early nursing-practice experiences. The first part of this chapter reflects the ways that students reacted to sometimes prolonged, difficult and emotionally draining situations with patients. The second part picks up on the students' experiences of what they saw as less-than-good care and describes some of the ways they dealt with them. Becoming hardened to the sometimes difficult things one is confronted with as a nurse is an often-discussed notion in nursing. I wondered what students felt about the concept.

Aspects of emotional labour

Alice described how she felt exposure to patients as a nurse affected the way she thought about caring.

> **Alice**: Maybe caring is being affected by what happens to others; we're taught not to take it home with you: leave it at work. But how can you be a caring person and not go home and think about somebody you've left, who you've been with for eight hours? You can't detach yourself from somebody you've been intimate with for eight hours ... sat at the side of the bed or done intimate things to or with and cared for ... You can't just cut off from that. Your working life is part of your life; so, whatever happens, whatever interactions you have with anybody, it affects you ... It is difficult to cut off.

Here Alice points out the difficulty she finds in cutting off from possible difficulties at work. It appears that there is a personal cost from investing emotion in a patient interaction. Here she describes the ways in which nursing affects her.

> **Chris**: Does your nursing affect you that much?
> **Alice**: I often have a few tears.
> **Chris**: How do you feel about that?
> **Alice**: I think it shows you are a caring person.

Alice seems to believe that to care properly one needs to be affected. Joan had also found things difficult at times.

> **Joan**: I think there is a big difference between hardness and being able to bottle up your emotions until there is an appropriate time to let it all out. I

think hardness, you know, that's basically being desensitized or something, and when you do that you don't treat the person as a person.

Chris: How do you mean?

Joan: You kind of keep yourself at a distance. And really that's not a caring nature, not to me it isn't anyway. I mean, it's more like ... treating the person as a disease itself rather than actually a person. But I do think you need to control your emotions to a certain extent. Otherwise ... all the nurses would just cry at every opportunity, and you know, how's that going to make the patients feel? So maybe that's why I started feeling a bit ashamed because of the fact that I actually started crying when I was in the room and I was saying goodnight.

Chris: What happened?

Joan: I started crying outside the room, because I just couldn't help but let it all out. But that's how I felt at the time anyway. It was also my ... first near-death kind of an experience, you know, with a patient; that kind of made things hard.

Joan's experience of caring with new and harrowing situations shows something of the difficulty of caring for patients, at times, especially for newcomers to nursing. She describes the need to cover or hide her emotions to protect the patient. This view is echoed in Wong et al.'s (2001) study, in which nurses described avoiding patients with terminal illness in order to protect themselves, an action that would not help the patient understand or come to terms with their diagnosis and prognosis. Hochschild (1979) considers that nurses do not suppress emotion in the full sense of the word. Instead, they shape it. It may be, as students, they have not fully developed this ability to shape the potent emotions evoked in the caring process, creating stress and feelings of personal sadness.

Students move around quite a lot in their training programmes and are exposed to many new care situations; not all are happy or easy to deal with.

Dealing with sub-optimal care: the students' perspective

Carrying forward the theme from the previous chapter, we pick up on some of the difficulties some students face when dealing with the realities of patient care. Carl had experienced situations that seemed to upset him, particularly at times when he did not have enough time to do all he wanted to do for the patients.

Chris: Have you seen things in nursing that you don't feel happy with?

Carl: Yeah, I have seen examples where ... I wonder if that's defensible in a caring role. I suppose I might have been guilty of it myself ... when you walk onto a very busy ward, for example, when there is a lot of pressure in various ways being placed on the individual nurse, then ... the defence is that we're only human and that we have our limitations.

Chris: What other things do you find upset you?

Carl: OK, well I mean I've seen examples of, say, nursing staff who really give the individual patients the very minimum access to their time, that they perform the task or the clinical operation procedure that is required and basically that is it – don't go beyond that; also the use of rather abrupt language as well. That makes me sad.

Joan too had observed examples of what she considered as being poor or sub-standard care from the more senior staff.

Joan: I was talking to an elderly gentleman and he was just finishing his dinner. The nurse was doing the drug round. Each patient has a little locker behind the bed. She got the appropriate drugs out and [was] obviously going to give it to him. He was saying about the dinner, making small talk; he wasn't feeling too good at the time, and he wanted to say, 'I have eaten my dinner', and she goes, 'Oh, sorry. What was that?' And he goes, 'I have eaten my dinner', and she goes, you know, 'Here, here take this tablet' ... She didn't listen at all to what he said and I could just look at his face and I can imagine what that could be like. It's not nice to be snubbed like that. And by somebody just doing a minor thing like that it can really make the person feel low and insignificant ... But then, having said that, I've seen nurses that don't do that, you know, who have a lot of communication: they have a good chat and have a good laugh and that.

Jess, the second-year student nurse, also commented on her experiences of difficult situations while caring.

Jess: There has been something that has upset me. I did actually see someone being verbally abusive to quite an elderly person. ... The patient was quite verbally abusive in themselves, but I didn't think that the way this nurse reacted was professional. It really did upset me ... I didn't feel in a position to be able to tackle them about what this person had said. But I did offer the patient some comfort afterwards, once the nurse had gone.

Here we can see how hard it is for junior, student nurses to intervene and point out that they are not happy with sub-standard care. This can add to the emotional burden experienced by students. Not everyone feels that they can take risks, especially students.

Anton is a third-year student nurse; he too had witnessed what he perceived as poor care and poor attitudes from more experienced nurses.

Anton: They don't seem to negotiate or talk with patients who might have confusion or other conditions. For example, an elderly person starts losing all their faculties and there's a staff nurse who says things like, he's a such and such, do you understand what I mean? They suppose I expect too much from them. They don't respond to the individual; they respond to the behaviour. For example, somebody is buzzing to go to the toilet or they are in distress or they don't sympathize with them. Straight away they judge it; they put a label on that patient.

Anton is clearly very upset by the ways he sees some of his more senior colleagues react towards certain patients. It is hard for students to speak up in the ward setting. Anton described some of the ways he controlled his emotion when he was upset.

> **Anton**: I think I can manage. I can take my emotions away and put them somewhere in a drawer.

Students often face terminal illness and sometimes death in their patients, often for the first time during the early part of their training period. Paula, a third-year student, had done one of her educational placements in a hospice specializing in the care of terminally ill patients in her first year.

> **Paula**: I've not actually been with anybody who's died, but I've seen them in their last days before they've died ... I think it's worse if you've become close to them and you've got to know them, or you know that they've not ... got any close relations or family. I think that's difficult [because then] the nurse probably needs to take on the role and develop a relationship with the patient.

Paula felt that making time for the patient was essential; again she too had seen instances that she did not feel comfortable with. She described a situation where she was not sure how to express her emotional feelings.

> **Paula**: I don't like to see a nurse rushing and in a hurry to move patients about ... as if they're not there or as if the task is more important than the patients. I really don't like that. If, say, they've got a number of jobs to do, and I realize that they've only got a short space of time, but ... they should make time for the patients. I mean, it's part of the role.
>
> **Chris**: You were saying you weren't sure if you needed to hide your emotions or let them all out. What did you mean by that?
>
> **Paula**: I think you do need to suppress them to an extent ... until a suitable time.
>
> **Chris**: Why?
>
> **Paula**: Because you don't want to project negative emotions onto your patients; it'll make them worse.

Paula unwittingly echoes Hochschild's (1979) and Bolton's (2000) views perfectly. She did not feel able to express her deep feelings of sadness or disappointment in her more senior colleagues. She felt that to be sad or to react in a normal way might be to harm her patients in some way. The first time she had discussed her upsetting experience had been with me. It is important to talk about these difficult situations. Adequate support systems need to be in place not just for students but also for more experienced staff as well. If we see the use of channelled or controlled emotion with patients as what Bolton (2000) calls a gift, it is clear that all involved in the nursing profession must ensure that support is available to all of the givers involved in care, particularly the new ones.

Conclusion

The concept of emotional labour has become a subject of importance in nursing, as it affects those whose job it is to care for patients (Phillips 1996). The effects of emotional labour probably affect all nurses; however, this study identified student nurses as being particularly susceptible to its influence. This view is supported by Allcock and Standen (2001), who point out that the relatively low status of students places them in a particularly difficult position and with little real support.

It is certainly the case that educationalists are actively promoting the philosophy of holism and individuality to students of nursing; however, as Henderson (2001) points out, it is unlikely that the same teachers are adequately preparing students for the strong emotions that this approach to care may bring. This is of clear concern as it is important to nurture newcomers to the profession of nursing. If students experience sadness and emotional trauma that is unresolved or buried, even in part, there may be a danger that they leave nursing altogether or may not later develop the caring attributes necessary for high-quality nursing care. As James (1989) writes, 'Emotional labour is hard work and can be sorrowful and difficult. It demands that the labourer gives personal attention ... not just a formulaic response.'

Despite the difficulties of dealing with the emotional demands outlined above, research shows that it is the satisfaction of working with and caring for patients which is still the reason for entering nursing (While 1998). I feel, however, that it is important to remain aware of these psychological assaults on the students' ability to cope with difficult emotional situations. As stated above, support should be provided for all nurses and healthcare providers. For nurses, it should be in the form of clinical supervision in the ward environment (Bassett 1999), and, for students, support and discussion of these issues should be a routine part of the education programme carried out by nurse lecturers in the comparatively safe environment of the classroom setting. Without this support, as Phillips (1996) points out, emotional labour may have far-reaching consequences for both caregivers and receivers.

CHAPTER ELEVEN

Summing it all up

Introduction

This book only considers the views and expressed beliefs of a relatively small selection of nurses and students, and, while interesting and valuable, it may not indicate what all patients may need or want. However, it has sought to highlight the issue of care as an important component of nursing practice. This importance has been explored and reinforced by the experiences of the nurses retold in this book.

This exploration has allowed the nurses to state personal views of their caring roles as nurses; in doing so it has provided many important insights into some of the ways in which they provide care for their patients. In addition to these very valuable insights, the study has also provided a glimpse of the rich contextual fabric of each person's nursing life.

Comparison of the findings with the literature

The literature has been used in a number of ways throughout this work. The themes that emerged from the research itself are present throughout the literature and, generally, the findings are compatible with the literature as it stands; however, occasionally the findings are new and striking. This book has been written to make clearer the beliefs of nurses and students in relation to their role in the nursing process. In revealing these views, many aspects of care have been identified and explored. The findings and expressed beliefs of the nurses clearly underline and reinforce the very complex nature of the phenomenon that we call 'care'. I will now compare the themes and identify where they appeared in the literature.

Aspects of making a connection

'Making a connection' was the first theme that emerged from the expressed sentiments of the nursees interviewed. This theme comprised five subcategories: 'making contact', 'tuning in', 'getting involved', 'being there' and 'humour'. The expressed feelings, attitudes and beliefs described ways of caring that epitomize the perceived closeness that is considered essential by the nurses in caring for their patients. 'Making a connection' is strongly linked to the nurses' ability to listen, comfort and express their sensitivity to patients.

Aspects of encouraging autonomy

The chapter entitled 'Encouraging autonomy' considered the notion of 'empowerment in patient care'. It was seen as an issue of importance to the nurses in this study. It was the only theme that did not contain subcategories, suggesting perhaps its strength as an underpinning value for nurses.

Aspects of giving of oneself

Caring is the essence of giving of oneself. This theme consisted of the subcategories 'using skills and knowledge', 'hands on' and 'the physical and emotional aspects of care'. Nurses give their time, energy and effort, and continue to spend time learning the skills and gaining the knowledge, both as students and as practitioners, necessary for providing high-quality care for patients. It would seem from the interviews that there are two quite distinct levels of care that they give to patients. They described not just the provision of physical care but also the giving of something of themselves. Here, perhaps, was described a depth of emotional benevolence or commitment provided for the patients. To simply provide mechanical care may not be enough in their eyes; providing care without genuineness was not seen as adequately caring for their patient.

Aspects of taking risks

This theme comprised the subcategories 'getting a buzz' and 'challenge'. Taking risks in nursing was associated with pushing the boundaries of accepted care. It was about moving from the defined boundaries of the profession and developing new and innovative ways of caring for patients.

Aspects of supporting care

This theme comprised the subcategories 'caring for colleagues', 'commitment' and 'ideals'. The respondents identified that there are certain essential factors required to ensure that care can be delivered effectively, that is, the importance of support systems, both managerial/organizational and psychological, of work. Coulon et al.'s (1996) and Fagerberg and Kihlgren's (2001) studies refer to this notion of support structures.

Aspects of emotional labour

This theme was unique to the students in this study; it reflected the – at times intense – emotional difficulties associated with learning to nurse. This concept was not identified in the more experienced nurses' interviews, that is to say that it is not an insignificant factor to them, just one that was not referred to. 'Emotional labour' used here is a term that describes the often very difficult things that nurses sometimes are expected to do in their daily work.

Congruence of findings to the literature

Now that the book is complete, it is important to assess the relationship between the findings and the evidence found within the literature. As evidenced above, there are strands throughout the literature that link strongly with the views and attitudes as expressed by the nurses in the study. In a sense, this is reassuring; it validates, at least in one way, that the research might be trustworthy. In terms of the themes 'making a connection', 'encouraging autonomy', and 'giving of oneself', there is a strong correlation between the interpreted, expressed words and the literature. The findings have a close match with other recent and influential studies (cited throughout this book) on the ways that nurses and patients see caring.

Closer examination of the studies in the literature shows that there are still some significant variations between what patients see as important and what nurses see as important. This is also true of the nurses in this text, as their expressed views seem to mirror previous studies in several important ways. This suggests nurses need to be very cautious about implementing strategies of care that they feel will enhance the patient experience. Before they implement anything, nurses need to be quite happy that the patients want them implemented. This, of course, makes clear the imperative need for more exploration into the relationship between nurses' perceptions of what constitutes good care and patients' perceptions of good care.

Moving on to consider the other themes of 'taking risks' and 'supporting care', their presence in the literature is much less well represented. My own view is that nurses do need to innovate and implement change in their practice. There is a trend for nurses and, indeed, other healthcare professionals to make both small and large changes in current practice. However, with this is associated the risk of stepping from the norm, the risk of challenging other more dominant healthcare professional groups, the obvious one being medicine, and also challenging managers and even academics; this needs considerable courage and strength from nurses wishing to make changes.

'Supporting care' appears to be associated with nurses who have developed a more managerial or organizational role within the caring environment. The issues surrounding the need for effective management systems that streamline communication and decision-making are clearly expressed in the views of some of the nurses. Leading on from this, and in fact closely related to it, both the experienced nurses and the students in the research place great value on psychosocial support.

'Commitment' and 'ideals' are considered as important to nursing, though are rarely mentioned by many of the nurses (that is not to say that the others do not have commitment and ideals). When referred to, however, they were seen as very important, although possibly leading to some frustration if other members of the team did not share them to the same levels. The students seemed to be strongly affected by emotional stress at times, and place great value upon support by more senior colleagues. This thread is closely related to the next theme, 'emotional labour'.

'Emotional labour', a theme unique to the students, was about the difficulty that some of the students found when dealing with emotional assaults placed upon them during their care for their patients. This seemed to be caused by their being unable to deal with distressing situations and also, significantly, from instances that students were witness to, and to what they saw as 'poor care' being delivered by the more senior and experienced nurses.

Future study

The feelings of the nurses in this book are illuminating and provide insight into how some nurses and students understand their role in the caring process. It is hoped that the book may stimulate further study into the related areas of caring. Apart from the obvious insights into nurses' and students' understanding of care and caring, there has been shown a great deal of material that describes the context of nursing itself. There are several areas that future researchers might wish to develop and pursue as a direct result of reading this book. These include the following.

- A further study exploring the expressed views of patients, enabling further comparison with the expressed views of the nurses in this study. One possible way to research this would be to use the subcategories and themes from this study to inform a semi-structured interview of a group of patients to search for common ground. Then, by using interpretive phenomenology in a similar way, to develop themes from the patients, thus providing further valuable insight into the patients' individual beliefs and conceptualization of their care.
- As some of the nurses' experiences in this book have shown, there are times when nurses have to, or should, adapt or deviate from, caring protocols to give patients necessarily individualized care. This should not be seen as taking a risk but as the appropriate reaction to the challenges facing healthcare today. Nursing can only move on if the other forces at play in healthcare allow it to. Research must be carried out to better understand the issues in order that barriers can be identified and overcome.
- 'Supporting care' is another area in which research could provide greater insights into the issues at play. As the NHS is encouraged to modernize, it may be argued that the systems in place that manage and control it are unable to support the absolute requirement that the ethos of high-quality care is supported as part and parcel of the structure of care in the NHS. In addition to the overarching structure required, it is also considered essential that individual nurses are supported via systems of counselling and clinical supervision, thus enabling them to maintain their initial commitment and ideals in caring for their patients. Research in this area would again help better identify such areas that need attention.
- Perhaps most importantly, this book has revealed something of the emotional stress that nursing students face in practice. It is important to ensure that this is explored more fully, to understand the effects that this might have on the long-term health and ability of the student (and later, qualified) nurse to continue to provide the care that our future patients need and deserve in the NHS and healthcare system in general.

Implications for practice

This book does not provide us with the definitive and absolute truth about care, caring and the ways that nurses understand and provide that care. What it does do, however, is provide much greater understanding and insight into what it is to care as a nurse or student nurse. It is hoped that managers, students, teachers and most importantly of all practising nurses will read this book and, in doing so, think more deeply about the ways they provide care for their patients and support their colleagues, be it as teachers of care, managers of care, or as actual providers of care.

Implications for society

Nursing, it is accepted, is an important part of any healthcare system throughout the world. What this book has shown are some of the ways that nurses care for their patients. The nurses interviewed spoke of the ways that they strive to make connections with their patients and of being there for them. They speak of encouraging greater independence in their patients and their patients' families, so that they become full partners in care, to enable them to have a deeper involvement in the caring process. They speak of the giving of something of themselves to the patients, in order that the patients can receive the significant benefits from nurses' skills and knowledge. They describe the ways that they put themselves on the line and take risks to improve the services that they can provide for patients. Finally, the nurses, and the students in particular, describe the emotional pressure and pain they feel in caring for the patients. All of these factors show, I believe, the great value that nurses and nursing represent to the patients in need of timely and highly expert nursing care.

Implications for education

This text has also shown the ways that some nurses and students understand care; it is clear that it has implications to educators of nursing. The main issues, as I see them, are related to the identification of care as being at the centre of the nursing curriculum. I believe that care has begun to be pushed from that position by various forces in recent years. I feel it important to reaffirm care as being of great importance to nursing. It really does need to be placed centre stage, not just by merely being referred to in lectures but also by the identification of the need for real support for practitioners of nursing and students alike. Teachers need to remember what it is like to begin to learn to nurse and, in doing so, help students to cope better with the severe emotional assaults that do occur when entering nursing.

Personal implications

Writing this book has been hard work, time-consuming and, at times, exasperating; however, it has also been extremely exciting and always very, very interesting. It has been a real privilege to speak with the nurses and students who took part in this project. In addition, the experience of speaking to the nurses will certainly enhance my teaching both in terms of content and in the way that I understand and relate to students and practitioners currently involved in nursing. They have provided me with many insights that have made me laugh and also feel really sad and very concerned at times. The expressed feelings and beliefs have, however, always impressed me with their honesty. I have also been highly impressed with the ways they have described how they have always tried to put the patients first in their care. One hears, unfortunately quite often today, that nurses don't care like they used to; this I believe to be untrue, at least in the nurses I had the privilege to interview in writing this book.

If this group is representative of other British nurses and students, I feel that nursing care is definitely present in British healthcare. It is important for policymakers at all levels to accept that nurses want to care for their patients. In order to do this, government, educationalists and managers, and nurses themselves, need to put the structures into place that will enable this to happen. This is needed for the sake of the patients that, after all, all of us have the potential to become.

As seems appropriate, the last word goes to a first-year student nurse, Alice.

Chris: Why did you want to become a nurse?

Alice: Because I like people. I love working with people. I think it enriches my life, working with other people. I can't ever envisage not working amongst people and interacting with people. I find that really satisfying.

Chris: Yes. But why nursing, because you could interact with people in lots of jobs, can't you?

Alice: I think it's that actually being involved in that therapeutic part of it, actually the doing of something rather than just, I don't know, interacting; I think feeling that you're doing something and making a difference.

The nurses' biographical details

The qualified nurses

Jack's story
Gender: Male
Area of practice: Education
Job title: Nursing lecturer
Qualifications: Registered nurse, BSc(Hons) nursing
Time qualified: 9 years

Jill's story
Gender: Female
Area of practice: Theatre
Job title: Staff nurse
Qualifications: Registered nurse
Time qualified: 2 years

Anne's story
Gender: Female
Area of practice: Theatre/education
Job title: Lecturer-practitioner, clinical co-ordinator
Qualifications: Registered nurse, Bachelor in Medical Science(Hons)
Time qualified: 15½ years

Lynn's story
Gender: Female
Area of practice: Day surgery
Job title: Staff nurse
Qualifications: Registered nurse, BSc(Hons)
Time qualified: 15 years

Sue's story
Gender: Female
Area of practice: Recovery
Job title: Staff nurse
Qualifications: Registered nurse, midwife
Time qualified: 14 years

Jackie's story
Gender: Female
Area of practice: General practice
Job title: Practice nurse
Qualifications: Registered nurse, midwife
Time qualified: 12 years

May's story
Gender: Female
Area of practice: ENT, ophthalmology, maxillo/facial
Job title: Acting ward manager
Qualifications: Registered nurse
Time qualified: 8 years

Pat' story
Gender: Female
Area of practice: General practice
Job title: Practice nurse
Qualifications: Registered nurse, midwife
Time qualified: 12 years

Cathy's story
Gender: Female
Area of practice: Mental health
Job title: Practice development adviser/lecturer, mental health
Qualifications: Registered mental nurse, MA
Time qualified: 11 years

Mike's story
Gender: Male
Area of practice: Oncology
Job title: Lecturer in oncology
Qualifications: Registered nurse, Master of Medical Science
Time qualified: 17 years

Steve's story
Gender: Male
Area of practice: ICU
Job title: Intensive-care staff nurse/lecturer
Qualifications: Registered nurse, BSc(Hons)
Time qualified: 6 years

Carla's story
Gender: Female
Area of practice: PACU
Job title: Lecturer/practitioner
Qualifications: Registered nurse, BA(Hons)
Time qualified: 14 years

Mary's story
Gender: Female
Area of practice: PACU
Job title: Sister
Qualifications: Registered nurse
Time qualified: 10 years

Jane's story
Gender: Female
Area of practice: Theatre
Job title: Staff nurse
Qualifications: Registered nurse
Time qualified: 22 years

Ingrid's story
Gender: Female
Area of practice: ENT
Job title: Staff nurse
Qualifications: Registered nurse, BSc(Hons)
Time qualified: 7 years

The students

Alice's story
Year of training: First
Gender: Female
Age: 34

Carl's story
Year of training: First
Gender: Male
Age: 43

Jess's story
Year of training: Second
Gender: Female
Age: 35

Joan's story
Year of training: Second
Gender: Female
Age: 23

Paula's story
Year of training: Third
Gender: Female
Age: 22

Anton's story
Year of training: Third
Gender: Male
Age: 31

References and further reading

Allcock N, Standen P (2001) Student nurses' experiences of caring for patients in pain. International Journal of Nursing Studies 38: 287–295.

Alligood MR (1992) Empathy: the importance of recognising two types. Journal of Psychosocial Nursing 30: 15–17.

Allmark P (1995) Can there be an ethics of care? Journal of Medical Ethics 21: 19–24.

Asrdt-Kurki P, Isola A (2001) Humour between nurse and patient, and among staff: analysis of nurses' diaries. Journal of Advanced Nursing 35(3): 452–458.

Ballie L (1996) A phenomenological study of the nature of empathy. Journal of Advanced Nursing 24: 1300–1308.

Barker P (2000) Reflections on caring as a virtue ethic within an evidence-based culture. International Journal of Nursing Studies 37: 329–336.

Barr W, Bush H (1998) Four factors of nurse caring in the ICU. Dimensions of Critical Care Nursing 17(4): 215–223.

Bassett C (1994a) Socialisation of student nurses into the qualified nurses' role. British Journal of Nursing 2(3): 179–82.

Bassett C (1994b) Nurse teachers' attitudes to research: a phenomenological study. Journal of Advanced Nursing 19(3): 585–592.

Bassett C (1995) Critical-care nurses: ethical dilemmas – a phenomenological perspective. Care of the Critically Ill 11(4): 166–169.

Bassett C (1996) Ethical problems in nursing the terminally ill. European Journal of Palliative Care 2(4): 166–168.

Bassett C (1999) Clinical Supervision: A Guide for Implementation. London: NT Books.

Bassett C (2001) Educating for care. Nurse Education in Practice 1: 2.

Bassett C (2002) Nurses' perceptions of care: a phenomenological study. International Journal of Nursing 8(8): 8–15.

Bassett C (in press) Defining care. Scandinavian Journal of Caring Science.

Beck CT (1994) Phenomenology: its use in nursing research. International Journal of Nursing Studies 31(6): 449–510.

Beck CT (1999) Quantitative measurement of caring. Journal of Advanced Nursing 30(1): 24–32.

Benner P (1984) From Novice to Expert. Menlo Park, CA: Addison-Wesley.

Benner P (1985) Quality of life: a phenomenological perspective on explanation, prediction and understanding in nursing. Advances in Nursing Science 8(1): 1–14.

Benner P, Wrubel J (1989) The primacy of caring: stress and coping in health and illness. Menlo Park, CA: Addison-Wesley.

Berman L (1988) Dilemmas in teaching caring: an outsider's perspective. Nursing Connections 1(3): 5-11.

Bertero C (1999) Caring for and about cancer patients: identifying the meaning of the phenomenon 'caring' through narratives. Cancer Nursing 22(6): 414-420.

Bolton S (2000) Who cares? Offering emotion work as a 'gift' in the nursing labour process. Journal of Advanced Nursing 32(3): 580-586.

Brycynska G (1997) Caring: The Compassion and Wisdom of Nursing. London: Arnold.

Bush H, Barr W (1997) Critical care nurses' lived perceptions of caring. Heart & Lung: The Journal of Acute & Critical Care 26(5): 387-398.

Campbell A (1994) Dependency: the foundational value in medical ethics. In Fulford K, Gillet GR, Soskie JM (eds.) Medicine and Moral Reasoning. Cambridge: Cambridge University Press.

Castledine G (1998) The relationship between caring and nursing. British Journal of Nursing 7(14): 866.

Cheung J (1998) Caring as the ontological and epistemological foundations of nursing: a view of caring from the perspectives of Australian nurses. International Journal of Nursing Practice 4: 225-233.

Chinn P (1985) Debunking myths in nursing theory and practice. Image 17(2): 45-49.

Chipman Y (1991) Caring: its meaning and place in the practice of nursing. Journal of Nursing Education 30(4): 171-175.

Clayton J (1999) Caring makes a difference. AORN Journal 70(6): 1059-1060.

Cohen J (1993) Caring perspectives in nursing education: liberation, transition and meaning. Journal of Advanced Nursing 18: 621-626.

Cohen MZ (1987) An historical overview of the phenomenologic movement. Image 19(1): 31-34.

Colaizzi PF (1978) Psychological research as the phenomenologist views it. In Valle R, King M (eds.) Existential-Phenomenological Alternatives for Psychology. New York: Oxford University Press.

Cormack DFS (1991) The Research Process in Nursing. Oxford: Blackwell Science.

Coulon L, Mok M, Krause K, Anderson M (1996) The pursuit of excellence in nursing care: what does it mean? Journal of Advanced Nursing 24: 817-826.

Crossley N (1996) Intersubjectivity. London: Sage.

Denzin NK, Lincoln YS (1994) Handbook of Qualitative Research. Beverly Hills, CA: Sage.

Drew N (1989) The interviewer experience as data in phenomenological research. Western Journal of Nursing Research 11(4): 431-439.

Dickoff J, James P (1986) Caring as perceived by the nursing profession. In Eddins B, Riley-Eddins E (1997) Watson's Theory of Human Caring: The Twentieth Century and Beyond. The Journal of Multicultural Nursing and Health 3(3): 30-35.

Dillon R, Stines P (1996) A phenomenological study of faculty-student caring interactions. Journal of Nursing Education 35(3): 113-117.

Dingman S, Williams M, Fosbinder D, Warnick M (1999) Implementing a caring model to improve patient satisfaction. Journal of Nursing Administration 29(12): 30-37.

Dyson J (1996) Nurses' conceptualisations of caring attitudes and behaviours. Journal of Advanced Nursing 23: 1263-1269.

Eddins B, Riley-Eddins E (1997) Watson's theory of human caring: the twentieth century and beyond. The Journal of Multicultural Nursing and Health 3(3): 30–35.

Ellis L (2001) Commonly used research methods. In Bassett C (ed.) Implementing Research in the Clinical Setting. London: Whurr Publishers Ltd.

Eriksen T (1992) Changing Patterns of Care. Copenhagen: Munksgaard.

Eriksson K (1992) The alleviation of suffering: the idea of caring. Scandinavian Journal of Caring Science 2: 119–123.

Eyles M (1995) Uncovering the knowledge to care. British Journal of Theatre Nursing 5(9): 22–26.

Fagerberg I, Kihlgren M (2001) Registered nurses' experiences of caring for the elderly in different health-care areas. International Journal of Nursing Practice 7: 229–326.

Fagerstrom L, Eriksson K, Engberg IB (1998) The patient's perceived caring needs as a message of suffering. Journal of Advanced Nursing 28(5): 978–987.

Field PA, Morse JM (1985) Nursing Research: The Application of Qualitative Approaches. Beckenham, Kent: Croom Helm.

Fletcher J (1997) Do nurses really care? An agenda for higher education following recent mergers. Journal of Nursing Management 5(3): 97–104.

Flick U (1999) An Introduction to Qualitative Research. London: Sage.

Gadamer H-G (1989) Truth and Method. Edited by Weinsheimer J, Marshall DG. New York: Crossroad.

Gaut D (1983) Development of a theoretically adequate description of caring. Western Journal of Nursing Research 5(4): 313–324.

Gaut D (1993) A vision of wholeness for nursing. Journal of Holistic Nursing 11(2): 164–171.

Gay S (1999) Meeting cardiac patients' expectations of caring. Journal of Advanced Nursing 18(4): 46–50.

Geekie S, Grieve A (1997) Caring amidst technology. Kaitiaki: Nursing New Zealand 3(2): 13–15.

Giorgi A (2000) The status of phenomenology in caring research. Scandinavian Journal of Caring Science 14: 3–10.

Gordon S (1991) Fear of caring: the feminist paradox. American Journal of Nursing 9(12): 45–48.

Gramling L, Nugent K (1998) Teaching caring within the context of health. Nurse Educator 23(2): 47–51.

Grams K, Kosowski M, Wilson C (1997) Creating a caring community in nursing education. Nurse Educator 22(3): 10–16.

Green AJ, Holloway DG (1997) Using a phenomenological research technique to examine student-nurses' understandings of experiential teaching and learning: a critical review of methodological issues. Journal of Advanced Nursing 26: 1013–1019.

Greenhalgh J, Vanhanen L, Kyngas H (1998) Nurse caring behaviours. Journal of Advanced Nursing 27: 927–932.

Grigsby K, Megel M (1995) Caring experiences of nurse educators. Journal of Nursing Education 34(9): 411–418.

Guba E, Lincoln Y (1995) Effective Evaluation: Improving the Usefulness of Evaluation. San Francisco, CA: Jossey Bass.

Halldorsottir S, Hamrin E (1997) Caring and uncaring encounters within nursing and health care from the patients' perspective. Cancer Nursing 20(2): 120–128.

Hankela S, Kiikkala I (1996) Intraoperative nursing care as experienced by surgical patients. AORN Journal 63(2): 435–442.

Hanson LE, Smith MJ (1996) Nursing students' perspectives: experiences of caring and not so caring interactions with the faculty. Journal of Nurse Education 35(3): 105–111.

Hare R (1981) Moral Thinking: Its Levels, Method and Point. Oxford: Oxford University Press.

Healy J (2000) Nursing stress: the effects of coping strategies and job satisfaction in a sample of Australian nurses. Journal of Advanced Nursing 31(3): 681–688.

Heidegger M (1962) Care beyond measure. In Moustakas C (1994) Phenomenological Research Methods. London: Sage.

Henderson A (2001) Emotional labor and nursing: an under-appreciated aspect of caring work. Nursing Inquiry 8(2): 130–138.

Higgins B (1996) Caring as therapeutic in nursing education. Journal of Nursing Education 35(3): 134–136.

Hochschild A (1983) The Managed Heart: Commercialisation of Human Feeling. Berkeley, CA: University of California Press. In Staden H (ed.) (1998) Alertness to the needs of others: a study of the emotional labour of caring. Journal of Advanced Nursing 27: 147–156.

Hochschild A (1979) Emotion work, feeling rules, and social structure. American Journal of Sociology 85: 551–575.

Hughes L (1995) Teaching caring to students. Nurse Educator 20(3): 3–5.

Hugman R, Peelo M, Soothill K (1997) Concepts of Care: Developments in Health and Social Welfare. London: Edward Arnold.

Holloway I, Wheeler S (2000) Qualitative Research for Nurses. Oxford: Blackwell Science.

Holstein J, Gubrium J (1994) Phenomenology, ethno-methodology and interpretive practice. In Denzin N, Lincoln Y (eds.) Handbook of Qualitative Research. London: Sage.

Jacox A, Bausell B, Mahrenholz D (1997) Patient satisfaction with nursing care in hospitals. Outcomes Management for Nursing Practice 1(1): 20–28.

James N (1989) Emotional labour: skill and work in the social regulation of feelings. Sociological Review 37: 15–42.

James N (1992) Care = organisation + physical labour + emotional labour. Sociology of Health and Illness 14(4): 488–509.

Jasper M (1994) Issues in phenomenology for researchers of nursing. Journal of Advanced Nursing 19: 309–314.

Jensen K (1993) Care: beyond virtue and command. Health Care for Women International 14: 345–354.

Jolley M, Brycynska G (1993) Nursing Care: The Challenge to Change. Sevenoaks, Kent: Edward Arnold.

Keane-McDermott S, Costain B, Rudisill K (1987) Caring: nurse–patient perceptions. Rehabilitation Nursing 12: 182–187.

Kelly D (1998) Caring and cancer nursing: framing the reality using selected social science theory. Journal of Advanced Nursing 28(4): 728–736.

Kincey J, Kat B (1984) How can nurses use social psychology to study themselves and their roles? In Skevington S (ed.) Understanding Nurses. Chichester: J Wiley & Sons.

Kincheloe JL, McLaren PL (1994) Rethinking critical theory and qualitative research. In Denzin N, Lincoln Y (eds.) Handbook of Qualitative Research. London: Sage.

Kirk JL, Miller M (1986) Reliability and Validity in Qualitative Research. Beverly Hills, CA: Sage.

Kirkevold M (2000) Qualitative methods in the caring sciences: time for critical reflection and dialogue. Scandinavian Journal of Caring Science 14: 1–2.

Knacck P (1984) Phenomenological research. Western Journal of Nursing Research 6(1): 107–114.

Koch T (1994) Establishing rigor in qualitative research: the decision trail. Journal of Advanced Nursing 19: 967–986.

Komorita N, Doehring K, Hirchert P (1991) Perceptions of caring by nurse educators. Journal of Nursing Education 30(1): 23–29.

Kosowski MMR (1995) Clinical learning experiences and professional nurse caring: a critical phenomenological study of female baccalaureate nursing students. Journal of Nurse Education 34(5): 235–242.

Kosowski M, Grams K, Wilson C (1997) Transforming cultural boundaries into caring connections. Journal of Nursing Science 2(6): 83–96.

Kovner CT (1989) Nurse–patient agreement on outcomes after surgery. Western Journal of Nursing Research 1: 7–19.

Kralik D, Koch T, Wotton K (1997) Engagement and detachment: understanding patients' experiences with nursing. Journal of Advanced Nursing 26: 399–407.

Kunyk D, Olson JK (2001) Clarification of conceptualisations of empathy. Journal of Advanced Nursing 35(3): 317–325.

Kyle TV (1995) The concept of caring: a review of the literature. Journal of Advanced Nursing 21(3): 506–514.

Lane JA (1987) The care of the human spirit. Journal of Professional Nursing 3: 332–337.

Larson PJ (1984) Important nurse-caring behaviours perceived by patients with cancer. Oncology Nursing Forum 11(6): 46–50.

Larson PJ (1986) Cancer nurses' perceptions of caring. Cancer Nursing 9(2): 86–91.

Larsson G, Peterson V, Lampic C, von Essen L, Sjoden P (1998) Cancer patient and staff ratings of the importance of caring behaviours and their relations to patient anxiety and depression. Journal of Advanced Nursing 27: 855–864.

Lauer P, Murphy S, Powers M (1982) Learning needs of cancer patients: a comparison of nursing and patient perceptions. Nursing Research 31: 11–16.

Lea A, Watson R (1996) Caring research and concepts: a selected review of the literature. Journal of Clinical Nursing 5: 71–77.

Lebold M, Douglas M (1998) Coming to know caring: a teaching learning journey. International Journal of Human Caring 2(1): 17–23.

Leininger M (1970) Nursing and Anthropology: Two Worlds to Blend. New York: John Wiley & Sons.

Leininger M (1977) Caring: The Essence and Central Focus of Nursing. The Phenomenon of Caring (part V). Kansas City, KA: American Nurses Foundation.

Leininger M (1978) Transcultural Nursing: Concepts, Theories and Practices. New York: John Wiley & Sons.

Leininger M (1981) The phenomenon of caring: importance, research questions and theoretical considerations. In Leininger M (ed.) Caring: An Essential Human Need. Thorofare, NJ: Slack.

Leininger M (1984) Care: The Essence of Nursing and Health. Thorofare, NJ: Slack.

Leininger M (1986) Care: facilitation and resistance factors in the culture of nursing. Topics in Clinical Nursing 8(2): 1–12.

Leininger M (1988a) Leininger's theory of nursing: cultural care diversity and universality. Nursing Science Quarterly 1(4): 152–160.

Leininger M (1988b) Ethnography and Ethno-nursing: Models and Modes of Qualitative Data Analysis. Qualitative Research Methods in Nursing. St Augustine, FL: Grune and Stratton.

Leinonen T, Leino-Kilpi H, Katajisto J (1996) The quality of intraoperative nursing care: the patients' perspective. Journal of Advanced Nursing 24: 843–852.

Lowenberg J (1993) Interpretive research methodology. Advances in Nursing Science 16(2): 57–69.

Lucke KT (1999) Outcomes of nurse caring as perceived by individuals with spinal cord injury during rehabilitation. Rehabilitation Nursing 24(6): 247–253.

Madjar I, Walton JA (1999) Nursing and the Experience of Illness. London: Routledge.

McGhee P (1998) RX: Laughter. RN 61(7): 50–53.

McKenna G (1993) Caring is the essence of nursing practice. British Journal of Nursing 2(1): 72–75.

McQueen A (1997) The emotional work of caring, with a focus on gynaecological nursing. Journal of Clinical Nursing 6(3): 233–240.

Morse JM, Bottorff JSM, Neander W, Solberg S (1991) Comparative analysis of conceptualisations and theories of caring. Image: Journal of Nursing Scholarship 23: 119–127.

Morse JM, Bottorff JSM, Hutchinson S (1994) The phenomenology of comfort. Journal of Advanced Nursing 20: 189–195.

Morse JM (1991) Comfort: refocusing of nursing care. Clinical Nursing Research 1(1): 91–113.

Moustakas C (1994) Phenomenological Research Methods. Beverly Hills, CA: Sage.

Natterlund B, Ahlstrom G (1999) Experience of social support in rehabilitation: a phenomenological study. Journal of Advanced Nursing 30(6): 1332–1340.

Norris CM (1989) To care or not to care – questions! questions! Nursing and Health Care 10(10): 545–547.

Nortvedt P (2001) Needs, closeness and responsibilities: an inquiry into some moral considerations in nursing care. Scandinavian Journal of Caring Science 2: 112–121.

Nursing and Midwifery Council (NMC) (2002) Code of Conduct. London: Nursing and Midwifery Council.

Oiler C (1982) The phenomenological approach in nursing research. Nursing Research 31(3): 178–180.

Paley J (2000) Husserl, phenomenology and nursing. Journal of Advanced Nursing 26: 187–193.

Parahoo K (1997) Nursing Research Principles, Process and Issues. London: Macmillan.

Pascoe E (1996) The value to nursing research of Gadamer's hermeneutic philosophy. Journal of Advanced Nursing 24: 1309–1314.

Petersson V, von Essen L, Sjoden PO (2000) Perceptions of caring among patients with cancer and their staff. Cancer Nursing 23(1): 32–39.

Phillips P (1993) A deconstruction of caring. Journal of Advanced Nursing 18: 1554–1558.

Phillips S (1996) Labouring the emotions: expanding the remit of nursing work? Journal of Advanced Nursing 24: 139–143.

Poole G, Rowat K (1994) Elderly clients' perceptions of caring of a home-care nurse. Journal of Advanced Nursing 20(3): 442–429.

Radsma J (1994) Caring and nursing: a dilemma. Journal of Advanced Nursing 20(3): 444–449.

Raatikainen R (1997) Nursing care as a calling. Journal of Advanced Nursing 25: 1111–1115.

Radwin L (2000) Oncology patients' perceptions of quality nursing care. Research in Nursing and Health 23(3): 179–191.

Ray M (1994) The richness of phenomenology, philosophic, theoretic, and methodological concerns. In Morse JM (ed.) Critical Issues in Qualitative Research. Beverly Hills, CA: Sage.

Rayman KM, Ellison GC, Holmes GE (1999) Towards a caring culture in professional nursing. Seminars for Nurse Managers 7(4): 188–192.

Reinharz S (1983) Phenomenology as a dynamic process. Phenomenology and Pedagogy 1(1): 77–79.

Riemen JD (1986) Non-caring and caring in the clinical setting: patients' descriptions. Topics in Clinical Nursing 8(2): 30–36.

Rittman M, Paige P, Rivera J, Godown I (1997) Phenomenological study of nurses caring for dying patients. Cancer Nursing 20(2): 115–119.

Roach SM (1987) The Human Act of Caring. Ottawa: Canadian Hospital Association.

Roach SM (1991) The call to consciousness: compassion in today's health world. In Gaut DA, Leininger MM (eds.) Caring: The Compassionate Healer. New York: National League for Nursing Press.

Robson C (1993) Real World Research: A Resource for Social Scientists and Practitioner Researchers. Oxford: Blackwell Science.

Roche J (1973) Phenomenology, Language and the Social Sciences. New York: Routledge.

Ryden MB (1998) A theory of caring and dementia. American Journal of Alzheimer's Disease 13(4): 203–207.

Sanford KD (2000) The competency of caring, leading with love. Surgical Services Management 6(6): 26–29.

Salvage J (1990) The theory and practice of the 'new nursing'. Nursing Times 86(1): 42–45.

Schultz A (1967) The Phenomenology of the Social World. Chicago, IL: Northwestern Press.

Schultz A, Bridgham C, Smith M, Higgins D (1998) Perceptions of caring. Clinical Nursing Research 7(4): 363–378.

Schoenhofer S, Boykin A (1998) Discovering the value of nursing in high-technology environments: outcomes revisited. Holistic Nursing Practice 12(4): 31–39.

Schoenhofer S, Bingham V, Hutchins G (1998) Giving of oneself on another's behalf: the phenomenology of everyday caring. International Journal for Human Caring 2(2): 23–29.

Scott PA (1995) Care, attention and imaginative identification in nursing practice. Journal of Advanced Nursing 21: 1196–1200.

Simonson C (1996) Teaching caring to nursing students. Journal of Nursing Education 35(3): 100–104.

Simpson S (1999) Holistic nursing – a return to healing. Creative Nursing 5(30): 16.

Smerke J (1990) Ethical components of caring. Critical Nursing Clinics of North America 2(3): 509–513.

Smith P, Barnes S, Jennings P (1998) The secret ingredient. Nursing Times 94(6): 34.

Smith M (1999) Caring and the science of unitary human beings. Advances in Nursing Science 21(4): 14–28.

Smith M, Sullivan J (1997) Nurses' and patients' perceptions of most important behaviours in a long-term care setting. Geriatric Nursing 18(2): 70–73.

Sourial S (1996) An analysis and evaluation of Watson's theory of human care. Journal of Advanced Nursing 24(2): 400–404.

Sourial S (1997) An analysis of caring. Journal of Advanced Nursing 26: 1189–1192.

Spiegelberg H (1960) The Phenomenological Movement: A Historical Introduction. The Hague: Nijhoff.

Sprengal A, Kelley J (1992) The ethics of caring: a basis for holistic care. Journal of Holistic Nursing 10(3): 231–238.

Staden H (1998) Alertness to the needs of others: a study of the emotional labour of care. Journal of Advanced Nursing 27: 147–156.

Stevens P, Schade A, Chalk B, Slevin O (1993) Understanding Research. Edinburgh: Campion.

Stevenson JS (1990) Quantitative care research: review of content, process, product. In Stevenson JS, Tripp-Riemer M (eds.) Knowledge About Care and Curing: State of the Art and Future Developments. Washington, DC: American Academy of Nursing.

Strauss A, Corbin J (1997) Grounded theory in practice. Beverly Hills, CA: Sage.

Sundin K, Axelsson K, Jansson L, Norberg A (2000) Suffering from care as expressed in the narratives of former patients in somatic wards. Scandinavian Journal of Caring Science 14: 16–22.

Swanson J, Chenitz W (1982) Why qualitative research in nursing? Nursing Outlook 4: 241–245.

Swanson KM (1991) Empirical development of a middle-range theory of caring. Nursing Research 40(3): 161–166.

Swanson KM (1993) Nursing as informed caring for the well-being of others. Image: Journal of Nursing Scholarship 25: 352–357.

Swanson KM (1999) What is known about caring in nursing science. Journal of Advanced Nursing 30(6): 1322–1331.

Swanwick M, Barlow S (1994) How should we define the caring role? Professional Nurse 9(8): 554–559.

Taylor B (1993) Ordinariness' in nursing: a study. Nursing Standard 7(29): 35–40.

Tennant S (1999) Nursing to care or caring to nurse: a qualitative investigation of perceptions of new recruits. Nurse Education Today 19: 239–245.

Thibodeau J (1993) Caring for a patient: a phenomenological enquiry. Nursing Outlook 14(1): 15–19.

Tournier P (1985) Creative Suffering. London: SCM Press.

Tschudin V (1986) Nursing: The Caring Relationship. London: Heinemann.

Tuck I, Harris L, Renfro T, Lexvold L (1998) Care: a value expressed in philosophies of nursing services. Journal of Professional Nursing 14(2): 92–96.

United Kingdom Central Council (UKCC) (1985) Code of Conduct. London: United Kingdom Central Council for Nursing and Midwifery.

Valentine KL (1991) Nurse–patient caring: challenging our conventional wisdom. In Gaut DA, Leininger MM (eds.) Caring: The Compassionate Healer. New York: National League for Nursing.

Van der Wal (1999) Furthering caring through nursing education. Curatonis: South African Journal of Nursing 22(2): 62–71.

Van Manen M (1990) Researching Lived Experience: Human Science for an Action Sensitive Pedagogy. New York: State University of New York Press.

Vincent J, Alexander J, Money B, Patterson M (1996) How parents describe caring behaviours of nurses in paediatric intensive care. American Journal of Maternal/Child Nursing 4: 197–201.

Von Essen L, Sjoden P (1991) Patient and staff perceptions of caring: review and replication. Journal of Advanced Nursing 16: 1363–1374.

Waddell D (1996) Why should we care? Georgia Nursing 56(5): 1.

Walsh M, Dolan B (1999) Emergency nurses and their perceptions of caring. Emergency Nursing 7(4): 24–31.

Walters AJ (1995) A hermeneutic study of the experiences of relatives of critically ill patients. Journal of Advanced Nursing 22: 998–1005.

Watson J (1979) Nursing: A Philosophy and Science of Caring. New York: Little, Brown and Company.

Watson J (1988) Nursing: Human Science and Human Care. New York: Appleton-Century-Croft.

Watson W (1999) Elderly patients' perception of care in the emergency department. Journal of Emergency Nursing 25(2): 88–92.

Webb C (1996) Caring, curing, coping: towards an integrated model. Journal of Advanced Nursing 23(5): 960–968.

Webb C (1995) What kind of nurses do patients want? Journal of Clinical Nursing 4(2): 101–108.

While A (1998) Reflections on nursing as a career choice. Journal of Nursing Management 6(4): 231–237.

Widmark-Petersson V, von Essen L, Sjoden P (2000) Perceptions of caring among patients with cancer and their staff. Cancer Nursing 23(1): 32–39.

Wilkes L, Wallis M (1998) A model of professional nurse caring: nursing students' experience. Journal of Advanced Nursing 27: 582–589.

Williams A (2001) A study of practising nurses' perception and experiences of intimacy within the nurse–patient relationship. Journal of Advanced Nursing 35(2): 188–196.

Williams SA (1998) Quality and care: patients' perceptions. Journal of Nursing Care Quality 12(6): 18–25.

Woodward VM (1998) Caring, patient autonomy and the stigma of paternalism. Journal of Advanced Nursing 28(5): 1046–1052.

Wolf Z, Colahan M, Costello A, Warwick F, Ambrose M, Giardino E (1998) Relationship between nurse caring and patient satisfaction. Medsurg Nursing 7(2): 99–105.

Wong F, Lee W (2000) A phenomenological study of early nursing experiences in Hong Kong. Journal of Advanced Nursing 31(6): 1509–1517.

Wong F, Lee W, Mok E (2000) Educating nurses to care for the dying in Hong Kong. Cancer Nursing 24(2): 112–121.

Yam B, Rossiter J (2000) Caring in nursing: perceptions of Hong Kong nurses. Journal of Clinical Nursing 9: 293–302.

Index

123